EXERCISE PRESCRIPTION

for Special Populations

Chronic Diseases, Unique Populations, and Challenging Diagnoses

Brian C. Leutholtz, PhD, FACSM

Professor
Department of Health, Human Performance, and Recreation
Robbins College of Health and Human Sciences
Baylor University
Waco, Texas

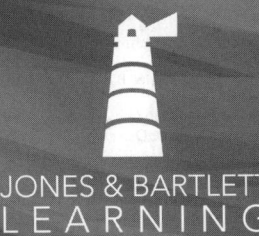

JONES & BARTLETT
LEARNING

World Headquarters
Jones & Bartlett Learning
5 Wall Street
Burlington, MA 01803
978-443-5000
info@jblearning.com
www.jblearning.com

Jones & Bartlett Learning books and products are available through most bookstores and online booksellers. To contact Jones & Bartlett Learning directly, call 800-832-0034, fax 978-443-8000, or visit our website, www.jblearning.com.

Production Credits

VP, Product Management: Amanda Martin
Director of Product Management: Cathy L. Esperti
Product Manager: Sean Fabery
Product Specialist: Andrew LaBelle
Project Manager: Jessica deMartin
Digital Project Specialist: Rachel DiMaggio
Director of Marketing: Andrea DeFronzo
VP, Manufacturing and Inventory Control:
Therese Connell

Composition: Exela Technologies
Project Management: Exela Technologies
Cover Design: Scott Moden
Media Development Editor: Troy Liston
Rights & Media Specialist: Rebecca Damon
Cover Image (Title Page, Section Opener):
© RaZZeRs/iStock/Getty Images Plus/Getty
Images
Printing and Binding: McNaughton & Gunn

Library of Congress Cataloging-in-Publication Data

Names: Leutholtz, Brian C., author.
Title: Exercise prescription for special populations : chronic diseases, unique populations, and challenging diagnoses / Brian C. Leutholtz.
Description: First edition. | Burlington, MA : Jones & Bartlett Learning, [2021] | Includes bibliographical references and index.
Identifiers: LCCN 2019041537 | ISBN 9781284180930 (paperback)
Subjects: MESH: Exercise Therapy—methods | Heart Diseases—therapy | Chronic Disease—therapy
Classification: LCC RM725 | NLM WB 541 | DDC 613.7/1—dc23
LC record available at https://lccn.loc.gov/2019041537

6048

Printed in the United States of America
24 23 22 21 20   10 9 8 7 6 5 4 3 2 1

To my good buddy and loyal companion, Ralph.

Brief Contents

Contents

SECTION 2   Other Common Chronic Diseases   57

Preface

▶ Purpose of This Text

Exercise Prescription for Special Populations: Chronic Diseases, Unique Populations, and Challenging Diagnoses was written to fill a void in the literature. The current textbooks addressing exercise prescription for special populations include discussions of chronic diseases within patient groups that are rarely, if ever, seen for exercise prescriptions by health professionals. The individual patients in these groups are typically capable of varying degrees of physical activity, making general, or "one size fits all," exercise guidelines nearly impossible to prescribe. Examples of such patient groups are those diagnosed with multiple sclerosis, muscular dystrophy, amyotrophic lateral sclerosis (ALS), mental illnesses, deafness, and blindness. This text, by contrast, focuses on how practitioners should prescribe exercise for those with conditions such as heart disease, diabetes, and hypertension, as well as for those who are pregnant, wheelchair dependent, or adolescent. These latter three populations are encountered by practitioners and personal trainers frequently, but they are often overlooked in the texts that are currently available.

Additionally, the texts utilized in the classroom today typically require a professor who is experienced in the field of exercise physiology to fully understand and elucidate the content, and they are typically written for clinically oriented graduate students or undergraduates majoring in exercise physiology or a related field. This text is still written for those students, but it also has been written for anyone in the health professions, such as nurses, doctors, personal trainers, dietitians, and exercise physiologists, and even patients. *Exercise Prescription for Special Populations: Chronic Diseases, Unique Populations, and Challenging Diagnoses* utilizes a hybrid approach, combining elements of a traditional textbook and a "field guide" reference. This reference aspect makes this text an ideal fit not just for students, but also for exercise physiologists and personal fitness trainers; the text is compact enough to be carried into an exercise environment or workout class, hospital, or cardiac rehabilitation program (both inpatient and outpatient). This text could also serve as a required or recommended resource for certification programs, such as those from the American Council on Exercise (ACE), the American College of Sports Medicine (ACSM), and many others. Furthermore, the current textbooks lack adequate supplemental resources for the classroom; this text includes a full suite of instructor resources, which are listed below.

Finally, this text reflects my 30 years of experience working and researching in clinical patient settings and with healthy populations, as well as writing some of the early guidelines adopted by the ACSM.

▶ The Structure of This Text

Each chapter of the text begins with an introduction designed to educate the health professional about the basics of the topic, including risk factors, warning signs, and general and background information. This is followed by a brief section on medications, discussing any that are relevant to the chronic disease and any that may impact the recommended exercise prescription. A subsequent section addresses any concerns and warning signs to watch out for. Specific exercise recommendations and exercise testing and evaluation guidelines are also covered in each chapter.

▶ How to Use This Text

This text includes the following features:

- **Learning Objectives** at the beginning of each chapter focus students on the key concepts of each chapter and the material that they will learn.

- **Quick-Reference Exercise Tables** summarize the exercise prescription for the special population by frequency, intensity, duration, modality, and warning signs. It can be used by the student, trainer, or healthcare professional during the supervision of an actual exercise session, or as a quick reference or reminder on the topic.

- **Patient Questions** consist of exercise and health questions commonly asked of healthcare providers or exercise physiologists prescribing and monitoring exercise relating to the special population. These "real-world" questions are included to help prepare students for working in the field, and to help the health professional better understand how the chronic disease affects the patient and his or her family life. It reflects many of the questions that patients have asked me over the years I spent working in rehabilitation and exercise programs, and will be useful when students, trainers, or healthcare providers work with and/or prepare to work with that particular patient group.

■ A collection of **Case Studies** has been included at the end of the text to test the knowledge of the student, trainer, or healthcare provider after reading the relevant chapter.

▶ Instructor Resources

Qualified instructors can request access to a full suite of resources, including the following:

■ Test Bank
■ Slides in PowerPoint format
■ Answers to Case Study Questions
■ Web Links to online videos and additional references

About the Author

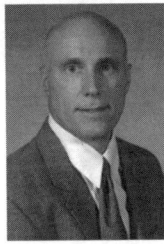

Courtesy of Baylor University.

Brian C. Leutholtz, PhD, FACSM, is a clinical professor working with students in the graduate and undergraduate program in exercise physiology at Baylor University in Waco, Texas. Dr. Leutholtz's role at Baylor has been to improve the graduate curriculum and complete the development of a PhD program by teaching and creating new graduate-level courses in sports nutrition and exercise prescription for special populations. He has previous experience as the director and founder of the Old Dominion University Therapeutic Exercise Program for Chronic Disease (TEMPO) in Norfolk, Virginia; has worked as a consultant for a managed care team providing exercise and diet evaluation and education in Virginia Beach; and served as the coordinator of the graduate program in exercise physiology at Baylor University. Prior to graduation in 1992 from Michigan State University, where he earned a PhD specializing in the study of clinical exercise physiology and cardiovascular physiology, Dr. Leutholtz completed a 4-year doctoral fellowship training program at Butterworth Hospital in Grand Rapids, Michigan, in clinical exercise physiology. As a fellow of the American College of Sports Medicine (ACSM), Dr. Leutholtz has earned recognition at the highest level of certification by the ACSM as a Clinical Program Director, and has recently added to his list of book publications a co-authored book entitled *Exercise Prescription: A Case Study Approach to the ACSM Guidelines, Second Edition*. In this book, the long-standing ACSM equations were improved, and a new term, the VO_2 *reserve*, was adopted by the ACSM.

Acknowledgments

The author and publisher would like to acknowledge the feedback provided by the following reviewers of the original manuscript proposal:

Phoebe Ajibade, EdD, MS
Associate Professor
Sport Science and Fitness Management Program
College of Health and Human Sciences
North Carolina A&T State University
Greensboro, North Carolina

Page Glave, PhD
Associate Professor
Department of Kinesiology
College of Health Sciences
Sam Houston State University
Huntsville, Texas

B. Sue Graves, EdD
Associate Professor and Director of the FAU Well Program
Department of Exercise Science and Health Promotion
Charles E. Schmidt College of Science
Florida Atlantic University
Boca Raton, Florida

Shannon L. Jordan, PhD
Assistant Professor
Department of Health and Kinesiology
College of Education and Human Development
Lamar University
Beaumont, Texas

Ryan Koenig, PhD
Assistant Professor and Program Director of Exercise Physiology
Exercise Physiology Program
College of Education and Human Performance
West Liberty University
West Liberty, West Virginia

Jordan Macht, PhD, CSCS
Lead Professor of Sport Medicine, Assistant Professor of Human Performance
Sport Medicine/Exercise Science Program
Division of Human Performance
College of Arts and Sciences
Campbellsville University
Campbellsville, Kentucky

Kelly Massey, PhD
Associate Professor and Clinical Coordinator of Exercise Science
Exercise Science Program
School of Health and Human Performance
College of Health Sciences
Georgia College and State University
Milledgeville, Georgia

Steven A. McCorkle, MS
Assistant Professor of Exercise Science
Kinesiology/Exercise Science Program
Department of Health and Kinesiology
College of Nursing and Health Sciences
Mississippi University for Women
Columbus, Mississippi

Braden Romer, PhD, CSCS
Assistant Professor of Exercise Science
Exercise Science Program
Department of Exercise Science
Congdon School of Health Sciences
High Point University
High Point, North Carolina

Dan Tarara, EdD, ATC, LAT, CES, SFS
Associate Professor and Department Chair
Exercise Science Program
Department of Exercise Science
Congdon School of Health Sciences
High Point University
High Point, North Carolina

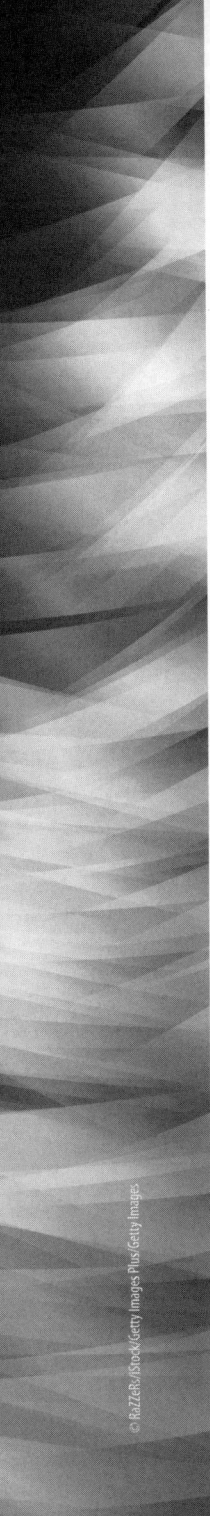

SECTION 1

Cardiovascular Disease

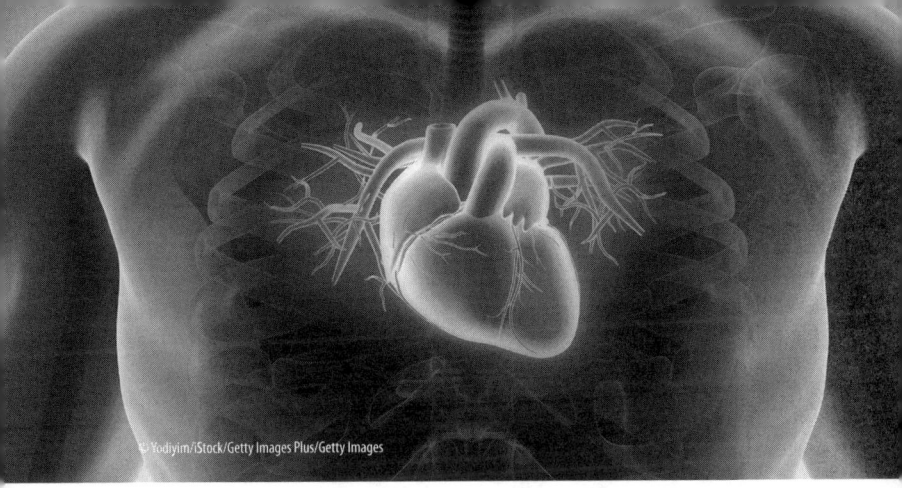

CHAPTER 1

Heart Disease: An Overview

LEARNING OBJECTIVES

Upon completion of this chapter, the reader will be able to:

- Understand the current medical philosophy in the United States.
- Identify the number one cause of death in the United States.
- Name the risk factors for heart disease.
- Explain the difference between arteriosclerosis and atherosclerosis.
- Understand the difference between angina and a myocardial infarction or "heart attack."
- Describe the different surgical procedures performed to treat heart disease.
- Identify and describe the different phases of cardiac rehabilitation.

The primary medical philosophy in America has been to cure disease. Interestingly, and somewhat ironically, by curing a disease, healthcare providers are intentionally trying to put themselves out of business. Only recently have healthcare providers started to look more into prevention for chronic diseases.

Heart disease is the major killer of Americans, and other diseases such as diabetes, obesity, cancer, and arthritis many times are associated with heart disease . It has been reported by the Centers for Disease Control and Prevention (CDC) that, in the United States, one of every four deaths is a result of heart disease. That is approximately one death every 38 seconds. Furthermore, approximately 92.1 million Americans have heart disease, which costs between 300 and 600 billion dollars each year!

Atherosclerosis, one of the causes of heart disease, is the process of plaque build-up in the arteries and other blood vessels. It develops slowly, beginning at an early age, and its significance is dependent upon many factors. Risk factors include things like age, family history, smoking, obesity, high blood pressure, elevated blood fats, and diabetes. Autopsies performed on American soldiers who served in World War II reported an alarmingly high prevalence of nonsignificant atherosclerosis, or plaque build-up, in the coronary arteries.

Another term associated with heart disease is arteriosclerosis. This term is frequently used interchangeably with atherosclerosis because the spelling and pronunciation are very similar. Arteriosclerosis is a hardening of the arteries that is most often present in older, more stable plaques in the arteries. This form of blood vessel problem can have consequences similar to atherosclerosis, resulting in heart attacks and increases in blood pressure.

Other terms frequently associated with heart disease are angina and myocardial infarction. Angina is chest pain, which results from a lack of oxygen delivery to the heart muscle when the heart is not receiving enough blood flow, and will be discussed in greater detail later. Unlike skeletal muscles, the heart muscle is much less tolerant of a lack of oxygen and can, therefore, become necrotic or die within an hour if treatment is delayed. It is important to understand that experiencing angina does not necessarily mean one is having a heart attack, but it is definitely a warning sign to get to a doctor. Stomach cramps, abdominal pain, and indigestion can be confused for angina, and vice versa. Always treat any pain in your chest and arm area as angina if there is any uncertainty. By going to the emergency room, doctors can rule out other causes by performing an electrocardiogram (ECG), blood work, and possibly other tests. True angina pain is typically deep, throbbing pain and pressure that is felt in the left arm and jaw. It also may be accompanied by nausea and sweating.

Myocardial infarction, or heart attack, is the actual blockage of an artery, and it may occur with or without angina. The blockage of the artery usually results when the plaque ruptures or explodes, creating jagged edges that attract blood platelets (fragments of blood cells involved in the clotting process). These platelets can adhere to the ruptured area and stop the flow of blood to the heart. As mentioned previously, the heart is a very aerobic organ; it requires a constant supply of oxygen or the tissues will begin to die. When blood flow (and oxygen) is interrupted, the heart muscle builds up lactic acid, which can disrupt its main energy source of fatty acids.

If a person does experience a myocardial infarction, a couple of treatments are typically done. Once the heart and patient have been stabilized, a cardiologist is usually the first doctor seen. He or she will decide whether to perform what is called a percutaneous coronary intervention (PCI), or refer the patient to a heart surgeon for coronary artery bypass surgery (CABS). If a PCI is performed, the cardiologist, working in a catherization (cath) lab, will attempt to open up the blocked vessel or vessels to restore blood flow to that region of the heart. The arteries most commonly treated are the left circumflex artery and the right coronary artery. Using a balloon catheter, the doctor will press the plaque against the wall of the blocked artery. If the procedure is successful, the doctor may place a wire-like device called a stent to help maintain the flow of blood and dramatically reduce the risk of restenosis, or the vessel "closing up," which may be as high as 30% without a stent. If the procedure is unsuccessful, or an artery such as the left main is blocked, the cardiologist may consult the surgeon for a CABS. Coronary artery bypass surgery is a much more invasive procedure that takes place in the operating room. There are newer and less-invasive methods; however, the details of these procedures are beyond the scope and intent of this book. In CABS, the saphenous vein in the lower leg is used to create the vessels or conduits needed to bypass the blocked artery. This vein can be dissected in numerous smaller sections, attached to the aorta, and used where needed to bypass the blockage in the heart. Another option is to use a chest artery, called the internal mammary artery. This vessel is left attached to the subclavian artery and detached from the chest area to be used to form a bypass. These artery grafts tend to remain free of plaque build-up or have a better patency when compared to vein grafts.

Following a heart attack, patients are often referred to a cardiac rehabilitation program. At this time, the patient will be given an exercise plan that should include the frequency, intensity, duration, and modality of exercise. Medications and cost/benefits also may be discussed.

Cardiac rehabilitation programs normally have four phases. Phase I involves inpatient acute care and lasts from a few days to several weeks, dependent on the number of complications. Phase I can be overwhelming to the patient, with visits from many different healthcare providers. Visits from the heart surgeon, cardiologist, nurses, dietitians, exercise physiologists, and social workers are commonplace. Things such as diet, exercise, and medications are usually the hallmark of this phase. A good understanding of medications and how they may affect the patient's exercise or target heart rate should be discussed, as some medications may adversely affect peak oxygen consumption; paradoxically, this may have a positive effect on blood pressure.

Ideally, the patient is referred and set up to attend Phase II: outpatient cardiac rehabilitation. Phase II usually lasts between 18 and 36 sessions (the length may be dependent on insurance reimbursement), with the goal to educate the patient to continue exercise on his or her own in the next phase. Unfortunately, as a result of patient scheduling conflicts, transportation, or unwillingness to attend, many patients do not move to the next phase. Those who do can expect to participate in sessions three days per week, typically on Mondays, Wednesdays, and Fridays, for 1 hour at the rehabilitation unit in the hospital. Here, they will encounter mainly nurses and exercise physiologists who will review their medications and monitor their blood pressure and target heart rate. Resistance training, typically with light dumbbells or circuit machines, also may be introduced as part of the exercise prescription, usually at an RPE (rated perceived exertion) intensity equivalent to the patient's aerobic target heart rate, or 30% to 50% of 1-RM (repetition maximum) (see Appendices A and B).

Originally, upon competition of Phase II, the patient continued to Phase III in the hospital, which was essentially the same as Phase II, and then to Phase IV, which was an off-site program. Currently, however, insurance companies are usually reluctant to pay for additional in-hospital programs and the patient is encouraged to transfer to an off-site program earlier in the process. Examples of off-site programs may include YMCAs, local gyms, walking groups, etc. Some of these off-site programs may even offer staff who are trained to occasionally check a blood pressure or other cardiac measure.

📝 PATIENT QUESTIONS

I am so young, why did I have a heart attack?
The process of plaque build-up begins at a very young age and
continues throughout life. Genetics and lifestyle play major roles in how
fast and how much plaque develops in your blood vessels as you age.

Why do I get chest pain?
Any chest pain is serious. Chest pain can occur when your heart is not
getting enough blood (and, therefore, oxygen). It does not always
mean that you are having a heart attack, but any chest pain should be
evaluated immediately if it is the first time you have experienced it or if
it is changing as it relates to your activity.

Why did my doctor do a stress test?
Your doctor did a stress test to see how your heart responds to exercise
or activity. Your heart rate was increased to approximately 85% of its
maximum to see if there were any signs or problems.

**My doctor did a heart catheterization. What exactly is the reason
for that?**
You may have had a positive stress test, so your cardiologist did a
catheterization under local anesthesia in the cath lab to evaluate which
blood vessels were blocked and what the extent of the blockage was.

Why did I need surgery?
If your catheterization revealed a blocked artery that could not be
opened, your doctor referred you to a cardiac surgeon for coronary
artery bypass surgery (CABS). In many instances, a blood vessel in your
leg is removed and used to do the bypass(es). After recovery, you can
be referred to a cardiac rehabilitation program.

**Do I need to go to cardiac rehabilitation? I feel much better and
my arteries are now fixed.**
By going to cardiac rehabilitation classes, you will learn how to exercise
to reduce the chances that you will have another heart attack. Topics
such as nutrition and many other related topics will be discussed.

Notes

_____

_____

_____

_____

_____

_____

_____

_____

_____

_____

_____

_____

_____

_____

_____

_____

_____

_____

_____

_____

_____

_____

_____

_____

_____

Notes

Notes

_____

_____

_____

_____

_____

_____

_____

_____

_____

_____

_____

_____

_____

_____

_____

_____

_____

_____

_____

_____

_____

_____

_____

_____

_____

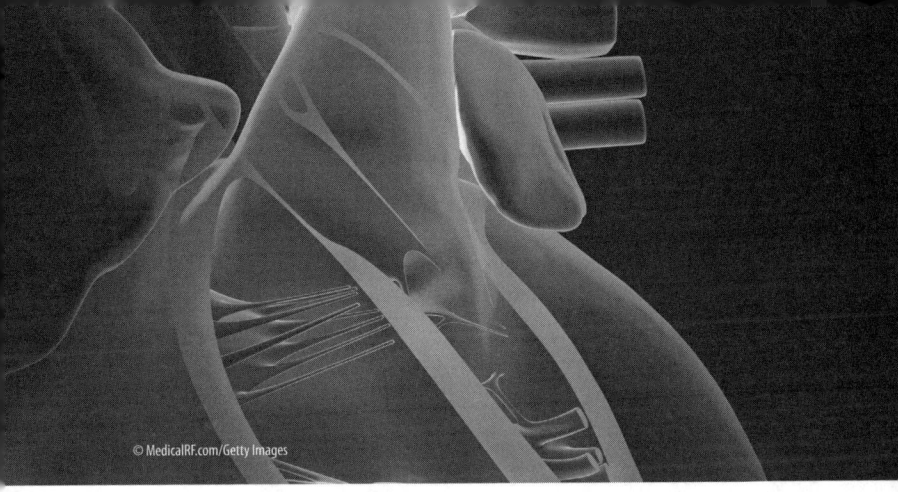

CHAPTER 2

Congestive Heart Failure

▶ **Introduction**

Congestive heart failure (CHF; also known as chronic heart failure) is a complex clinical syndrome that involves abnormal functioning of the left ventricle. Because the left ventricle is the stronger, pumping side of the heart, cardiac output—and, therefore, blood flow—can be seriously compromised. To further complicate this disease, abnormal neurohormonal regulators are affected, resulting in effort intolerance, fatigue, shortness of breath, exercise intolerance, fluid retention, and increased mortality and morbidity.

The term "downward spiral" has been used to describe CHF. It begins with low cardiac output. This triggers the body into compensatory reactions because the body believes that there is not enough blood flow for the organs and tissues. When this occurs, the sympathetic nervous system acts and compounds (renin-angiotensin) are released that constrict the blood vessels. Sodium and water retention (aldosterone release) result in additional fluid build-up in the lungs, ankles, and abdominal area. All of these factors work to increase the blood pressure and the workload on the heart, thus worsening CHF.

It has been estimated that five million Americans are in heart failure, with an estimated 200,000 new cases reported each year. The 5-year survival rate is 25% in males and 38% for females, and billions of dollars are spent each year treating CHF.

In right-sided heart failure, patients usually report fluid retention or swelling in their ankles and/or abdomen (called ascites). In left-sided heart failure, rales, which are produced by fluid build-up in the lungs, may be heard by auscultation with a stethoscope. A cough, tiredness, and shortness of breath (dyspnea or orthopnea) are typically reported to healthcare providers. The heart may be enlarged (cardiomyopathy) with a significant loss of viable myocardium tissue, which may have occurred from suffering a large myocardial infarction (heart attack). With only a 10% loss of viable heart tissue, the ejection fraction, a strong indicator of the heart's functionality, can drop below 50% (a normal ejection fraction being between 56% and 68%). As a result, many patients end up on a heart transplant list.

The heart may become so enlarged, a condition known as cardiomegaly, that idiopathic hypertrophic subaortic stenosis (IHSS) may result. This condition involves a large, hypertrophied left ventricle. The ventricular septum, a band of tissue separating the ventricles, may actually become so enlarged that it interferes with the aortic valve, further restricting cardiac output and worsening CHF.

Heart failure can have a variety of causes, including the following:

- Coronary artery disease
- Idiopathic (unknown cause)
- Hypertension
- Valvular problems
- Infections of the heart
- Alcohol and cocaine usage
- Inherited and/or congenital causes
- Malnutrition

▶ **Medications**

Medications used to treat CHF include digoxin and digitalis, which are tailored to help improve cardiac output and blood flow to the muscles and organs. Diuretics may be prescribed to reduce fluid build-up, while angiotensin-converting enzyme (ACE) inhibitors may help lower blood pressure and increase vasodilation. Beta-blockers may be recommended to reduce the stress on the heart. Some patients may receive a pacemaker if other therapies do not work.

▶ **Exercise**

Individuals with a history of CHF may have very low exercise capacities, reflected in ejection fractions in the 20s or 30s. Patients typically report early leg fatigue and a need to rest when returning home after a brief exercise session. Early fatigue may result from an increased dependence on fast-twitch (type II) muscle fiber recruitment, which elevates the levels of lactic acid in the muscles and blood. Exercise capacity can be improved by using peripheral adaptations such as increases in capillary densities, mitochondria, and slow-twitch (type I) fiber recruitment.

QUICK-REFERENCE EXERCISE TABLE: CONGESTIVE HEART FAILURE

Frequency	Intensity	Duration	Modality	Warning Signs
A minimum of 3–5 days per week of aerobic exercise	Rated perceived exertion (RPE) of 10–14 on the 6–20 scale	Interval/rest training may be necessary	Stationary cycle, rower, treadmill, or any other aerobic equipment deemed appropriate	A sudden weight gain of 3 or more pounds
Seven days per week may be prescribed provided patient is well-rested and motivated	A target heart rate can be prescribed between 100 and 140 beats per minute	Start with 5–10 minutes at the desired intensity, with rest periods of no more than twice the work minutes	Light hand weight exercises may be added once the patient has achieved 20 minutes of continuous supervised activity	Fluid retention in the ankles and/or swelling of the abdomen
Light hand-weights may be incorporated 2 days per week if desired	Intensity may need to be flexible based on patient's changing physical ability and medication (e.g., beta-blockers)	Try to achieve 20–45 minutes of continuous aerobic exercise	Swimming and aerobic dance classes may be appropriate once the patient has achieved 20 minutes of continuous supervised activity	An unusual cough, tiredness, and/or shortness of breath

📋 PATIENT QUESTIONS

Why is it important to monitor any weight gain I may have?
Any rapid or unexpected gain in your weight can signal a worsening of your CHF. You should contact your doctor if this occurs as soon as possible.

Why do I get tired so easily?
Your heart is not strong enough to pump enough blood to your muscles during activity. This will result in early fatigue and a burning or tight sensation in your leg or upper body muscles.

Will I ever be cured of my congestive heart failure?
CHF cannot be cured—it can only be treated with medications and positive lifestyle changes. At some point, you may need a heart transplant.

Why did I get congestive heart failure?
There are a number of reasons why you may have CHF, including having a large heart attack, inherited reasons, and/or lifestyle. Your doctor may know and be able to address the causes of your CHF.

Will I always be on medications?
Yes; your doctor may adjust your medication dosages from time to time, and may even recommend a pacemaker to help your heart pump better.

Why do I hear my doctor talking about something called my ejection fraction?
Your ejection fraction is a way to measure how well your heart is functioning. If it changes, your doctor may increase your medications and/or put you on a heart transplant list.

Notes

_____

_____

_____

_____

_____

_____

_____

_____

_____

_____

_____

_____

_____

_____

_____

_____

_____

_____

_____

_____

_____

_____

_____

_____

Notes

Notes

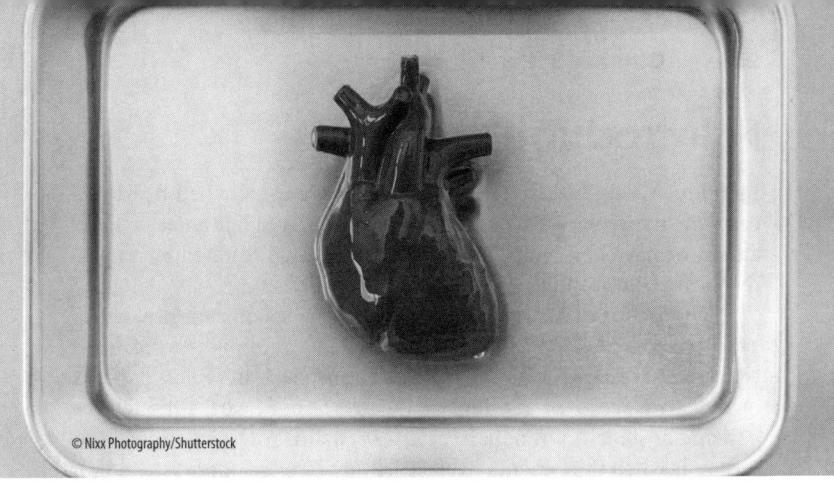

CHAPTER 3
Heart Transplant

LEARNING OBJECTIVES

Upon completion of this chapter, the reader will be able to:

- Identify the two main types of heart transplants.
- Describe the survival rates for patients with a heart transplant.
- List some absolute contraindications to heart transplant.
- Understand the important role medications have in preventing rejection.
- Explain and describe the unique challenges of prescribing exercise for heart transplant patients.
- Describe how to prescribe exercise intensity for a patient with a heart transplant.
- Understand how patients with a heart transplant increase their cardiac output during exercise.

▶ **Introduction**

Individuals who have a heart transplant have usually had heart disease for many years. Many have sustained a large left anterior heart attack, or have had multiple heart attacks, which resulted in congestive heart failure and the need for a transplant.

Thousands of heart and other organ transplants are performed every year in the United States. The most common type of heart transplant is known as an orthotopic transplant, in which patient's own heart is removed and replaced with a donor heart, although the patient's aorta and pulmonary arteries remain. A less-common procedure is when the patient's heart is left in place to support the donor heart; this type of transplant is called a heterotopic or "piggyback" transplant.

The first patient to receive a heart transplant was a 54-year-old man named Louis Washkansky. It was performed by Dr. Christiaan Barnard on December 3, 1967, at Groote Schuur Hospital in Cape Town, South Africa. The patient was able to occasionally walk and talk; however, he died soon afterward of pneumonia, only living for 18 days. Unfortunately, at the time of the surgery, the immunosuppressant drugs used to help fight off rejection were unsuccessful. As a result, future transplants were put on hold to allow for the advancement of immunosuppressant drugs. Philip Blaiberg received the third heart transplant in 1968 and lived for 19 months. Today, patients can live much longer, some even surviving 30 years or more. In fact, it has been estimated that the 1-year, 3-year, and 5-year survival rates for heart transplants are 84%, 77%, and 65%, respectively, with an average life expectancy of approximately 9–15 years. There are approximately 230 hospitals in the United States equipped to perform transplants, most located in or near large metropolitan areas. Most candidates have suffered massive heart attacks, presenting with enlarged hearts or cardiomyopathies, and have had congestive heart failure for years, often to the point of near death.

Absolute contraindications include but are not limited to factors such as age, human immunodeficiency virus infection, substance abuse, pulmonary hypertension, smoking, and active cancers. Once a patient is cleared for a heart transplant, he or she is put on a transplant list. However, the list is not first come, first served, where the person who is first on the list is next in line, so it can be a rollercoaster ride of stress for many patients. The list takes into consideration things like urgency, blood type, size of the donor's heart, and other variables for a correct match to the recipient. Recipients are required to live close to the hospital, and some may even move to a nearby location. Once contacted, the patient usually has a limited time to arrive at the hospital. The operation may take up to about 4 hours.

▶ **Medications**

One of the main concerns for transplant recipients is that the body will reject the new heart. It is especially important to have regular biopsy scores taken during the first year and less frequently thereafter. Medications to help prevent rejection, including cyclosporine, prednisone, and tacrolimus, will have to be taken for the rest of the patient's life. Side effects these medications include infections, hyperlipidemia, hypertension, weight gain, osteoporosis, renal dysfunction, and diabetes.

▶ **Exercise**

Prior to transplantation, many patients have endured prolonged periods of inactivity and a sedentary lifestyle. As a result, many are in a catabolic state, having sustained a loss of lean body mass and reduced aerobic capacity. Other factors affecting their exercise ability may be lung complications, hypertension, chronotropic incompetence, and left ventricular dysfunction. All of these factors contribute to a poor aerobic capacity, reduction in cardiac output, and lethargy.

Once a successful transplant is performed and the patient has recovered enough to begin activity, there are a few considerations that the exercise professional must take note of and consider when prescribing exercise. With the transplantation, much of the autonomic nervous system is lost and denervation of the myocardium occurs. Thus, the sympathetic and parasympathetic control on the heart are compromised. This results in a lack of chronotropism (the ability to increase the heart rate normally via the sympathetic branch of the autonomic nervous system) and a lack of bridling on the sinoatrial node, which has an intrinsic rate of approximately 100 beats per minute without parasympathetic bridling. This results in a high resting heart rate, often near 100 beats per minute. Thus, prescribing aerobic exercise by target heart rate may not be appropriate. Using the rated perceived exertion (RPE) chart or substituting the systolic blood pressure for heart rate in the Karvonen equation may be considered, especially if the patient continues to be hypertensive after transplantation. See Appendix A for a more detailed explanation of these methods.

Resistance training, when appropriate, should be a part of the exercise regimen. Due to the long-standing sedentary lifestyle most patients experience, this places them in a catabolic state, causing a lot of lean tissue loss. Furthermore, muscle and bone loss caused by some medications results in an increasing need to emphasize resistance training (see exercise table that follows).

Another factor to consider is the patient's ability to increase their cardiac output (CO), sometimes expressed in liters per minute. Because the product of heart rate (HR) and stroke volume (SV; the amount of blood pumped by the heart with each beat) determines the cardiac output ($HR \times SV = CO$), and because the patient's ability to increase heart rate is very reduced, this limits the aerobic capacity by as much as 60% to 70% compared to normal. As cardiac output plays a role in aerobic capacity (see Fick Equation), these patients typically tire easily and have a very low exercise capacity. However, during exercise, the cardiac output and stroke volume, and thus aerobic capacity, can increase even when heart rate increases are minimal. This can occur in several ways. First, the contraction of muscles during exercise can help pump blood to the heart, known as venous return or preload; thus, the heart muscle is stretched. This stretching helps the heart to contract more forcibly as a function of the Frank-Starling Law (e.g., the more one stretches a rubber band, the harder it snaps back), thus improving stroke volume and cardiac output. A second way the heart can increase stroke volume and cardiac output is by reacting to catecholamines. Hormones, such as epinephrine and norepinephrine, are released by the adrenal glands in response to physical or emotional stress. These hormones attach to beta receptors on the heart, resulting in a more forceful contraction.

Patients who have received a heart transplant can demonstrate a small, but abnormal, increase in heart rate. Consequently, a third, but mostly insignificant, mechanism to increase cardiac output in cardiac transplant patients is known as the Bainbridge or atrial reflex. Here, stretch receptors located in the heart sense an increase in venous pressure and blood flow to the heart. These stretch receptors react by sending signals to the brain and heart to increase heart rate, with little or no effect on stroke volume.

QUICK-REFERENCE EXERCISE TABLE: CARDIAC TRANSPLANT

Frequency	Intensity	Duration	Modality	Warning Signs
A minimum of 3–5 days per week of aerobic and resistance exercise	Rated perceived exertion (RPE) of 10–14 on the 6–20 scale, or systolic blood pressure replacing heart rate into the Karvonen equation, following the same intensity for resistance training	Interval/rest training may be necessary	Stationary cycle, rower, treadmill, or any other aerobic equipment deemed appropriate	Any sudden change in weight
Seven days per week may be prescribed provided patient is well-rested and motivated	A target heart rate is not appropriate due to denervation of the heart	Start with 5–10 minutes at the desired intensity, with rest periods of no more than twice the work minutes	For most patients, light hand weights will be appropriate at first; however, more aggressive resistance training may be prescribed depending on age and physical abilities	Fluid retention in the ankles and/or swelling of the abdomen
Light hand weights or more aggressive resistance training should be incorporated with each exercise session	Intensity may need to be flexible based on patients changing physical ability, age, and medication (e.g., beta-blockers)	Try to achieve 20–45 minutes of continuous exercise, with half the time devoted to resistance training	Other methods of less-supervised exercise, such as swimming and aerobic dance classes, may be appropriate	Flu-like symptoms

📋 PATIENT QUESTIONS

Now that I have a new heart, am I "cured" of heart disease?

Unfortunately, even though you have a "new" heart, you are not cured from heart disease. Think of heart disease as total body disease. Your new heart is still vulnerable to heart disease, and it can also become diseased. By following positive lifestyle changes, however, you can reduce the chances of your new heart getting sick.

Will I still have to see a heart doctor now that I have a "new" heart?

Yes, you will still need to have regular check-ups with your family physician and possibly your cardiologist or surgeon. Routine biopsy tests may need to be performed to make sure your heart is adapting to your body. Medication also may need to be periodically updated.

Do I have to take my medications the rest of my life?

Yes, the medications prescribed by your doctor will have to be taken the rest of your life; however, adjustments and replacement medications may be prescribed from time to time.

How long can I expect to live with my new heart?

A lot of this will depend on how well you behave! Following your healthcare provider's advice on good lifestyle habits is extremely important. You could live for many more decades.

Will the medications I take prevent me from rejecting my new heart?

The medications that you take to help with rejection may prevent rejection. You will need to see your doctor on a regular basis to be tested for signs of rejection.

Why doesn't my heart rate increase very much when I exercise or am active?

When you received your new heart, some of the nerves that control your heart rate were cut. Your heart can still increase the flow of blood by other mechanisms, but your heart rate will not increase as much as it did when you had your own heart.

Notes

_____
_____
_____
_____
_____
_____
_____
_____
_____
_____
_____
_____
_____
_____
_____
_____
_____
_____
_____
_____
_____
_____
_____
_____
_____
_____

Notes

_____

_____

_____

_____

_____

_____

_____

_____

_____

_____

_____

_____

_____

_____

_____

_____

_____

_____

_____

_____

_____

_____

_____

_____

_____

_____

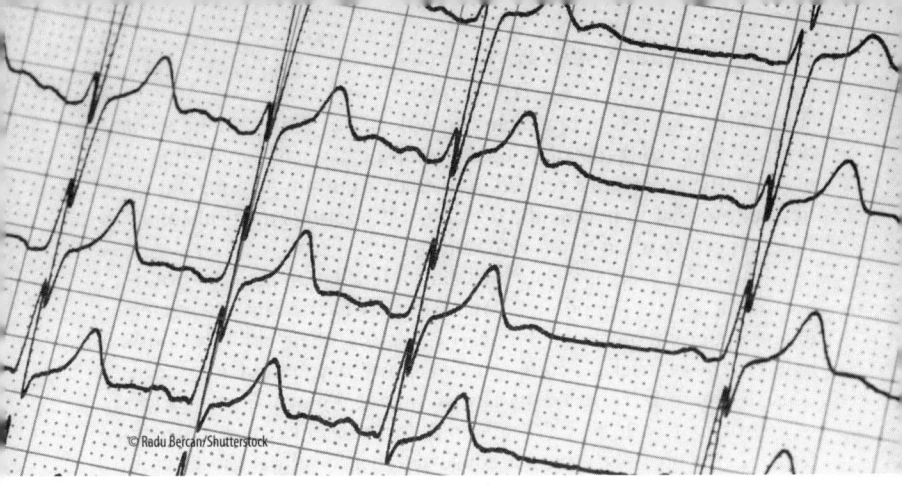
© Radu Bercan/Shutterstock

CHAPTER 4
Atrial Fibrillation

LEARNING OBJECTIVES

Upon completion of this chapter, the reader will be able to:

- Understand the pathophysiology and major risks of atrial fibrillation.
- Explain atrial kick and why it is important in atrial fibrillation.
- Explain the different treatments for atrial fibrillation.
- Explain how the frequency, intensity, duration, and modality of exercise should be individualized to each patient.

▶ Introduction

Atrial fibrillation is a common type of heart arrhythmia that can affect the people of all ages. Although it is not completely understood, it involves the sinoatrial (SA) node, or the pacemaker of the heart, and signals from the pulmonary veins firing erratically. These signals try to take over the job of the SA node. Atrial fibrillation can occur in an otherwise normal heart that is free of coronary artery disease or atherosclerosis. Patients usually report a fluttering or thumping in their chest with shortness of breath and weakness. The upper chambers of the heart (the atria) actually "quiver," resulting in a stasis or pooling of blood in the heart and a reduction in cardiac output. Although atrial fibrillation itself in not life threatening, it is a serious medical condition that can result in blood clots and stroke.

The major risks associated with atrial fibrillation include thromboembolic events (blood clots) and irregular heartbeats. As a result of the upper chambers of the heart quivering, their ability to push blood to the ventricles is compromised and cardiac output is reduced. This results in a reduction in cardiac output, known as atrial kick, of approximately 20%. This leads to a decrease in exercise capacity, fatigue, and possibly eventual congestive heart failure. Other concerns associated with atrial fibrillation include valvular disease, cardiomyopathies, hypertension, hyperthyroidism, and coronary artery disease.

▶ **Medications**

To treat atrial fibrillation, the goal is to return the heart's rate and rhythm to normal using one or more of the following methods, depending on the underlying cause and duration. The first method is called electrical cardioversion. Paddles or patches are placed on the chest; the heart is shocked and momentarily stopped. When it resumes, the hope is that it will be in a normal rhythm. If electrical cardioversion is successful, anti-arrhythmic medications, such as beta-blockers, amiodarone, digitalis, and verapamil, may be prescribed to prevent future occurrences of atrial fibrillation. Other, more-invasive procedures such as surgical or catheter ablation, may be performed. These procedures involve using surgery, radiofrequency, cryotherapy, or heat to scar the excited electrical pathways so that they cannot conduct electricity.

▶ **Exercise**

Exercise should be avoided until the atrial fibrillation is controlled under the supervision of a physician. Because the patient may be young or old, with or without coronary artery disease, the exercise prescription (i.e., frequency, intensity, duration, and modality) should be individualized to his or her specific needs and capacities.

QUICK-REFERENCE EXERCISE TABLE: ATRIAL FIBRILLATION

Frequency	Intensity	Duration	Modality	Warning Signs
A minimum of 3–5 days per week of aerobic and resistance exercise	Rated perceived exertion (RPE) of 10–15 on the 6–20 scale, or a target heart rate at an intensity between 50% and 85% of Karvonen (see Appendix A)	Interval/rest training may be necessary in older or deconditioned patients	Stationary cycle, rower, treadmill, or any other aerobic equipment deemed appropriate	Any sudden change in energy level; weakness and fatigue
Seven days per week may be prescribed, provided patient is well-rested and motivated	A target heart rate is not recommended if there are signs of an arrhythmia	Start with 5–10 minutes at the desired intensity, with rest periods of no more than twice the work minutes	For most patients, light hand weights will be appropriate at first; however, more aggressive resistance training may be prescribed depending on age and physical abilities	A fluttering or thumping in your chest, possibly accompanied by shortness of breath
Light hand weights or more aggressive resistance training can be incorporated with each exercise session	Intensity may need to be flexible based on patient's age and changing physical ability and medication (e.g., beta-blockers)	Try to achieve 20–45 minutes of continuous exercise at the prescribed target heart rate	Other methods of less-supervised exercise, such as swimming and aerobic dance classes, may be appropriate	Rapid weight gain or unusual chest pain

📝 PATIENT QUESTIONS

Why did I get atrial fibrillation? I have never suffered a heart attack.

Often, the cause of atrial fibrillation is unclear and serious complications are rare. Possible causes can be numerous and include high blood pressure, overactive thyroid, lung diseases, viral infections, stress, and many others.

Can my atrial fibrillation return?

Yes, it may return and your doctor may try another treatment. Be on the lookout for symptoms of a thumping in your chest and any unusual shortness of breath, weakness, and/or fatigue.

Will I always have to take medication for my atrial fibrillation?

Some of your medications may eventually be decreased or discontinued, whereas others you may have to stay on. Your doctor will monitor your heart and blood and decide the best course of action.

Am I likely to suffer a heart attack?

Atrial fibrillation can occur in otherwise healthy hearts free from coronary artery disease. If you exercise regularly and follow healthy lifestyle habits, you can reduce your chances of suffering a heart attack.

What happens if I do not take my medicine when my atrial fibrillation is "cured"?

Once you have a history of atrial fibrillation, it is more likely that it may return. If you are not taking your medicine, you may be more likely to have a blood clot lodge somewhere in your body, such as your brain, lungs, or heart.

My friend had atrial fibrillation and needed surgery. Will I need surgery?

If your atrial fibrillation is not controlled by medications and cardioversion, or keeps returning, a surgical method may need to be performed.

Notes

_____

_____

_____

_____

_____

_____

_____

_____

_____

_____

_____

_____

_____

_____

_____

_____

_____

_____

_____

_____

_____

_____

_____

_____

_____

_____

_____

Notes

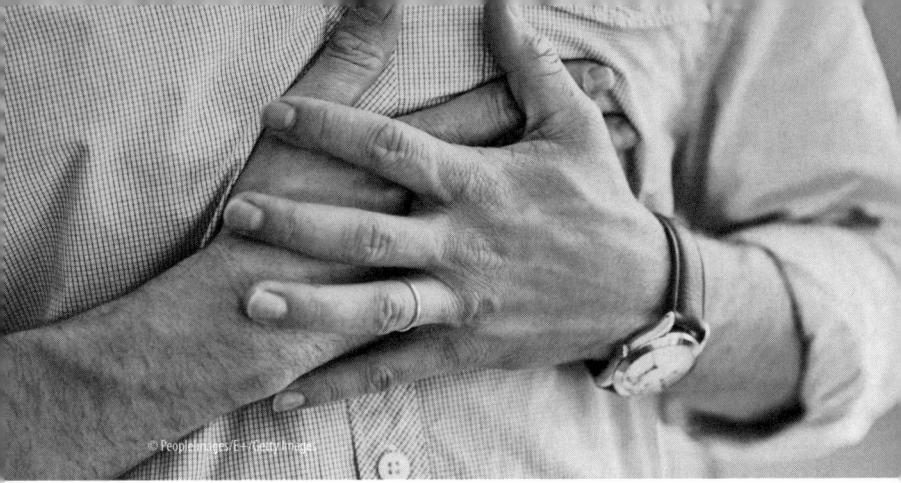

CHAPTER 5
Angina

▶ **Introduction**

Angina, or chest pain, is often confused with indigestion. It has been stated that "indigestion is the number one killer of Americans, not heart disease," because it is so often confused with true heart pain and not acted upon.

When the heart does not receive enough blood flow and oxygen, angina may result, which may lead to a myocardial infarction. Angina may occur at rest or during activity, and it may or may not result in a heart attack. In fact, only 50% of patients having a heart attack may experience the symptoms of angina. However, while it is important to make clear that angina may or may not mean that a heart attack is occurring, one should still seek the care of a hospital emergency room immediately when experiencing chest pain, regardless of the cause. Many patients describe angina in one or all of the following ways: "It was like an elephant was standing on my chest"; "I got all sweaty, short of breath, and nauseated"; or "There was a dull, achy pain in my jaw and left arm." If ever in doubt about whether the pain is indigestion or heart related, the patient should seek medical help immediately and go to the emergency room. When a patient reports to the emergency room, the main goal is to determine the true cause of the chest pain, to rule out a myocardial infarction. The patient will be hooked up to a heart monitor, and blood will likely be drawn to look for markers that would signify a myocardial infarction, such as specific cardiac enzymes and troponin. Other blood tests may be done to look for signs of inflammation, such as C-reactive protein and an enzyme named lipoprotein-associated phospholipase A2. Nitroglycerin, a medication that acts systemically on the body's blood vessels, also may be prescribed to see if it has an effect on reducing chest pain by opening up the blood vessels, a process known as vasodilation.

Angina is categorized into three main types. The first is called stable angina. This type of angina is predictable and may be associated with a patient's myocardial oxygen consumption, sometimes expressed as the rate pressure product (RPP), calculated as systolic blood pressure (SBP) × heart rate (HR). The RPP can be measured at the ischemic threshold, or the point at which angina may occur accompanied with ST-depression on the electrocardiogram (ECG). It may occur during certain activities when the heart is not getting adequate blood flow (e.g., climbing stairs or washing the car). Angina can usually be relieved with rest or nitroglycerin. It also may be the result of fixed or stable atherosclerotic plaque, likely to be present in older patients.

A second type of commonly reported angina is called unstable angina. Here, symptoms are less predictable; it may occur at rest and/or with low levels of physical exertion. With no baseline or predictability established, the first time that a patient experiences angina should fall into this category.

Prinzmetal's or variant angina is another type of angina. In Prinzmetal's angina, the patient may or may not have coronary artery disease, as the vessels may be free of significant obstruction. Vessel spasm or constriction usually occurs at rest, or even sleep, resulting in chest pain. Other factors that can trigger vessels to constrict are smoking; drug use; certain medications; trauma; rapid increases in blood pressure, as when lifting a heavy object; and possibly even catecholamines. Fire fighters who are startled or woken up suddenly when a fire alarm goes off in the middle of the night have reported this type of angina.

Outside of the three main types is walk-through angina; only one-tenth of 1% of people experience this type of angina. This type of angina can occur in both normal (disease-free) and atherosclerotic vessels. It involves mild angina during the first stages of exercise, followed by the disappearance of chest pain at higher workloads or myocardial oxygen consumptions. It is likely caused by the coronary arteries having a delayed response to vasodilatation. This type of angina may be difficult to reproduce in some patients with associated heart disease.

▶ Medications

Angina is typically treated with drugs designed to relax or open the heart's coronary arteries and increase the flow of blood and oxygen to the heart muscle. Medications such as beta-blockers, calcium channel blockers, ACE inhibitors or blockers, nitrates, and ranolazine may be prescribed. With the exception of beta-blockers, these drugs' effect on a target heart rate intensity is minimal. Cooldown periods following exercise may need to be extended to 10 minutes or more to prevent blood pooling in the lower extremities and dizziness. Hot showers or hot tub use may exacerbate vasodilation, and patients should be cautious to look for any signs of lightheadedness or dizziness.

▶ Exercise

The Canadian Cardiovascular Society's grading system is a commonly used way to grade angina. Angina is typically graded on a 1–4 scale.

With **Grade 1** representing the absence of angina with normal physical activity or activities of daily life, however with more strenuous activities, angina may present. Activities such as stair climbing, heavy meals, exposure to cold or hot ambient temperatures may cause **Grade 2** angina. **Grade 3** angina occurs when chest pain occurs at normal every day activities at home or at work. Finally, any type of physical activity apart from bed rest will result in angina and discomfort in **Grade 4** angina.

When prescribing exercise to a patient who may experience stable angina, it is important to know the ischemic threshold. The ischemic threshold is defined as the activity intensity where there is inadequate blood flow to the heart. This may result in angina or ST-segment depression on an ECG. Angina may not always occur at the same target heart rate intensity and the ischemic threshold may not always be at the same heart rate; it depends on the modality of exercise equipment and type of activity. Some types of activities can have a more isometric component compared to others, thereby having a greater effect on increasing the SBP. This could result in angina occurring at different heart rates on different types of equipment or when performing different exercises. For example, blood pressure can be higher during stationary cycling or arm ergometry compared to treadmill walking or jogging at a prescribed heart rate. The RPP should be measured and used as a guide for prescribing target heart rates; for example, an exercise target heart rate prescribed on the arm ergometer or for resistance training may be different when compared to the treadmill or rower. It is important for the healthcare provider to be aware of this and to understand that some target heart rates may not be appropriate for the anginal patient.

QUICK-REFERENCE EXERCISE TABLE: ANGINA

Frequency	Intensity	Duration	Modality	Warning Signs
A minimum of 3–5 days per week of aerobic and resistance exercise	Rated perceived exertion (RPE) of 10–15 on the 6–20 scale or a target heart rate at an intensity between 50% and 85% of Karvonen (see Appendix A)	Interval/rest training may be necessary in older or deconditioned patients	Stationary cycle, rower, treadmill, or any other aerobic equipment deemed appropriate	Any chest pain not normally associated with the activity
Seven days per week may be prescribed, provided patient is well-rested and motivated	Target heart rates may need to be specific to the exercise performed and should be based on the RPP and ischemic threshold	Start with 5–10 minutes at the desired intensity, with rest periods of no more than twice the work minutes	For most patients, light hand weights will be appropriate at first; however, more aggressive resistance training may be prescribed depending on age and physical abilities	Any sudden change in energy level; weakness and fatigue
Light hand weights or more aggressive resistance training can be incorporated with each exercise session	Intensity may need to be flexible based on patient's age and changing physical ability and medication (e.g., beta-blockers)	Try to achieve 20–45 minutes of continuous exercise at the prescribed target heart rate	Other methods of less-supervised exercise, such as swimming and aerobic dance classes, may be appropriate	Rapid weight gain or unusual chest pain

📋 PATIENT QUESTIONS

When I have chest pain, am I having a heart attack?
When you are having chest pain, your heart may not be receiving enough blood and oxygen. You should report it to your doctor or healthcare provider immediately and discontinue or reduce your activity until it disappears. If your chest pain occurs while under the supervision of a health professional, let that person know immediately.

Why can't my doctor "fix" my chest pain?
Your doctor is aware that you have chest pain. It may be that you have had the maximum number of bypasses possible or other surgeries. Your chest pain now may need to be treated with medicines.

What should I do when I think I feel angina?
If your angina is new, you are not sure it is angina, and/or it occurs during an activity not typically associated with chest pain, you should stop whatever activity you are doing and go directly to the emergency room.

Will I always have angina?
If you have had coronary artery bypass surgery and your doctor cannot perform any more bypasses, you may have to live with angina. If you have had a percutaneous coronary intervention, your doctor may recommend that you see a heart surgeon for a coronary artery bypass operation.

Will my medicine "cure" my angina so I will not have a heart attack or need surgery?
There are different types of medications that your doctor may put you on when you have angina and/or have a history of angina. Some medications can relax your blood vessels to relieve your angina, while others may be prescribed to lower your heart rate and reduce the stress on your heart. Medications cannot "cure" angina. Regular exercise and a proper diet will help to prevent angina from reoccurring.

Why do I sometimes feel angina when I exercise on certain types of exercise machines?
Some machines may have a greater isometric component, meaning that they may raise your blood pressure higher compared to other machines. Your blood pressure may play a role in angina. Let your healthcare provider or doctor know if you feel angina on any machines, as it might be that you should avoid that particular exercise machine or need to see your physician.

Notes

_____
_____
_____
_____
_____
_____
_____
_____
_____
_____
_____
_____
_____
_____
_____
_____
_____
_____
_____
_____
_____
_____
_____
_____
_____
_____
_____

Notes

_____

_____

_____

_____

_____

_____

_____

_____

_____

_____

_____

_____

_____

_____

_____

_____

_____

_____

_____

_____

_____

_____

_____

_____

_____

_____

_____

_____

_____

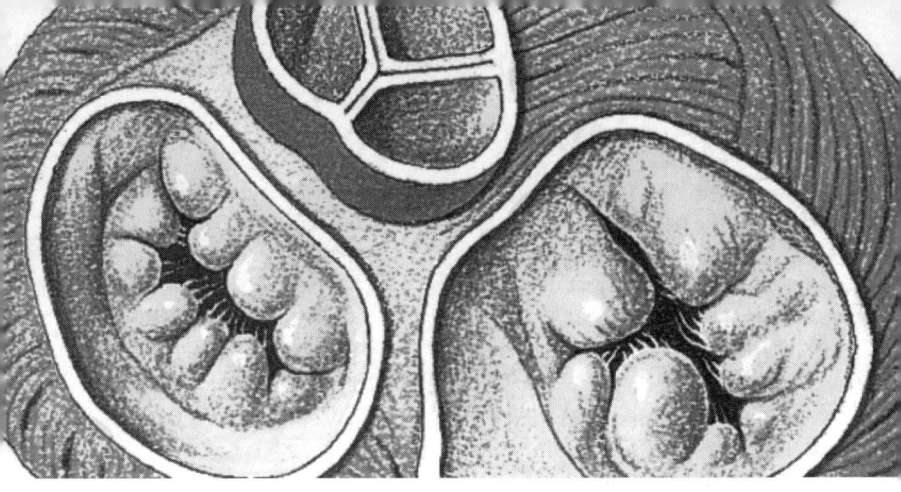

CHAPTER 6

Valvular Heart Disease

LEARNING OBJECTIVES

Upon completion of this chapter, the reader will be able to:

- List the symptoms of valvular heart disease.
- Name the four heart valves and provide their other associated names.
- Explain the difference between mechanical and tissue valves.
- Understand how damaged heart valves can be repaired.
- List and understand the typical medications that are prescribed to treat valvular disease and any effects they may have on the exercise prescription.
- Know in which types of valve disease exercise is contraindicated.

▶ **Introduction**

Patients who have valvular heart disease have damage to one of the four valves of the heart. Mild valvular disease may not have any symptoms, but in more severe cases, it may lead to congestive heart failure and possibly a heart transplant. Sometimes, even severe cases of valvular disease can go unnoticed. Patients of all ages can have valve problems. Valve problems may or may not be associated with atherosclerosis and/or myocardial infarction. Symptoms may include the following:

- Palpitations, chest pain (may be mild)
- Fatigue
- Dizziness or fainting (with aortic stenosis)
- Fever (with bacterial endocarditis)
- Rapid weight gain
- Heart failure
- Blood pressure changes

Common locations of valvular disease involve the mitral and tricuspid valves. The mitral valve is also named the bicuspid valve. It, along with the tricuspid valve, are known as the atrioventricular (AV) valves and they control the flow of blood between the atria and ventricles. The pulmonary valve is responsible for controlling the blood flow from the heart to the lungs. It also may be called a semilunar valve. Finally, another semilunar valve, the aortic valve, governs the flow of blood between the heart, aorta, and the rest of the body.

When valves become damaged, they can become narrow (stenotic), or they may not be able to open or close fully (known as incompetent). Often, the valve leaflets will prolapse and allow blood to flow backwards into the adjacent chamber, or regurgitate. Certain types of heart diseases are congenital, but many are acquired later in life. Rheumatic fever, bacterial infections of the heart, aging, certain medications, high blood pressure, radiation therapy, and a heart attack all may contribute to valvular heart disease. Aortic valve disease—a narrowing of the aortic valve, restricting the blood flow from the left ventricle to the aorta—is one of the more serious types of valve disease and may require valve repair or replacement.

Valve replacements are of two types: mechanical and tissue. A mechanical or manufactured valve is made of strong, durable materials designed to last the patient's lifetime. This type of valve is prone to attracting blood clots, which may lodge in the valve flaps or hinges. Therefore, a blood thinner is prescribed to the patient for the remainder of his or her life. Tissue valves, sometimes called bioprosthetic valves, are taken from animal donors. Tissue valves can last 10–20 years, and the patient may not need to be on blood thinners. A third, but less common, type of valve is a donor valve, which comes from a human donor.

Damaged heart valves can be repaired, but often are replaced. In many cases, the patient will be put on a heart-lung bypass machine and the chest and sternum opened. However, in some instances, a less-invasive surgery that still requires a heart-lung machine, called robotic mitral valve repair, may be performed to repair a valve and minimize trauma. This process involves a camera or endoscope and robotic arms controlled by the surgeon with hand controls and foot pedals. Only five small incisions on the right side of the chest are required to perform the surgery.

▶ Medications

Many of the medications to treat heart valve problems are commonly prescribed to treat high blood pressure and heart disease; they may include the following:

- ACE inhibitors
- Beta-blockers
- Antiarrhythmics
- Anticoagulants (blood thinners)
- Diuretics (water pills)
- Vasodilators
- Antibiotics
- Inotropes (digitalis)

▶ Exercise

Patients with mild valvular heart disease usually have few restrictions; however, with severe aortic valve disease or other serious valve conditions, patients need to be assessed by their physician before exercising. Some patients may require surgery before an exercise program can be safely prescribed. For postoperative patients, the program should include both aerobic and resistance training exercise. Keep in mind that the sternal incision may be sore and take additional time to heal. Some stretches focusing on this area may help with the stiffness and aid in recovery.

For younger or more active patients who wish to resume a more vigorous aerobic training schedule, such as marathon running or training, a maximal stress test is recommended to make sure everything looks stable.

QUICK-REFERENCE EXERCISE TABLE: VALVULAR HEART DISEASE

Frequency	Intensity	Duration	Modality	Warning Signs
A minimum of 3–5 days per week of aerobic and resistance exercise, if desired	Rated perceived exertion (RPE) of 12–16 on the 6–20 scale	Interval/rest training may be necessary in older or deconditioned patients	Stationary cycle, rower, treadmill, or any other aerobic equipment deemed appropriate	Any chest pain not normally associated with the activity
Seven days per week may be prescribed provided patient is well-rested and motivated	Target heart rate at an intensity between 50% and 85% of Karvonen (see Appendix A)	Start with 5–10 minutes at the desired intensity, with rest periods of no more than twice the work minutes	For most patients, light hand weights will be appropriate at first; however, more aggressive resistance training may be prescribed depending on age and physical abilities	Any sudden change in energy level; weakness and fatigue
Light hand weights or more aggressive resistance training can be incorporated with each exercise session	Intensity may need to be flexible based on patient's age and changing physical ability and medication (e.g., beta-blockers)	Try to achieve 20–45 minutes of continuous exercise at the prescribed target heart rate	Other methods of less-supervised exercise, such as swimming and aerobic dance classes, may be appropriate	Rapid weight gain or unusual chest pain

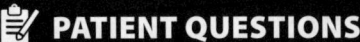

PATIENT QUESTIONS

How long will my heart valve last?
That depends on the type of heart valve your doctor gave you. If you have a tissue valve, it may last 10–20 years, while a mechanical valve may last you a lifetime.

Do I have to be careful when I exercise?
That depends on how active you were before your surgery. If you have had a previous heart condition, you should follow the exercise prescription given to you by a healthcare professional.

Will I always need to take my blood thinner?
If you have a mechanical valve, yes, you will be on the blood thinner for the rest of your life.

Why do I hear my heart valve "ticking" when I am sleeping or in a quiet place like my church?
You most likely have a mechanical heart valve and are probably more aware of the sound than those surrounding you.

My doctor told me that the blood vessels in my heart look normal and I have never had a heart attack. Why is that?
You can have a problem with your valve and still have normal blood vessels in your heart. Valve problems can occur in younger individuals free from heart disease.

Why does my dentist put me on an antibiotic before I go in for my appointment?
If you have an artificial heart valve, your heart may be at a greater risk for a bacterial infection. Your dentist may put you on an antibiotic to reduce your risk.

Notes

_____

_____

_____

_____

_____

_____

_____

_____

_____

_____

_____

_____

_____

_____

_____

_____

_____

_____

_____

_____

_____

_____

_____

_____

_____

_____

_____

_____

Notes

_____
_____
_____
_____
_____
_____
_____
_____
_____
_____
_____
_____
_____
_____
_____
_____
_____
_____
_____
_____
_____
_____
_____
_____

Notes

_____

_____

_____

_____

_____

_____

_____

_____

_____

_____

_____

_____

_____

_____

_____

_____

_____

_____

_____

_____

_____

_____

_____

_____

_____

_____

_____

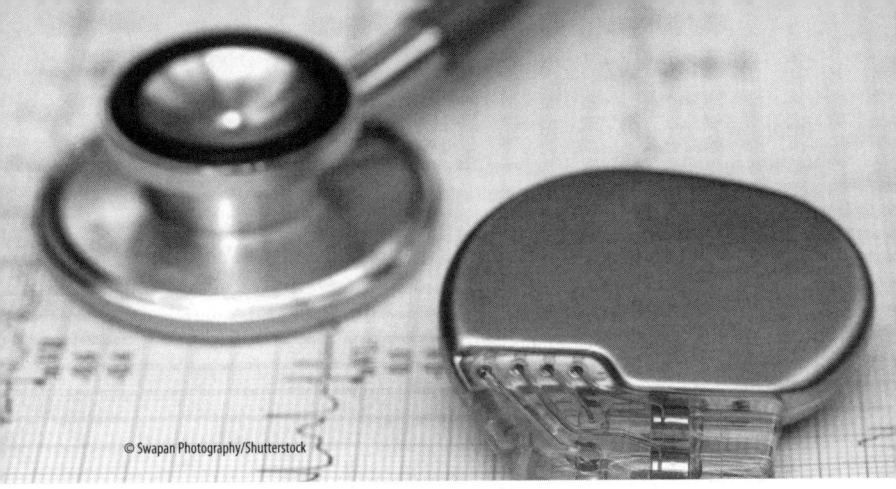

© Swapan Photography/Shutterstock

CHAPTER 7
Pacemakers

LEARNING OBJECTIVES

Upon completion of this chapter, the reader will be able to:

- Understand the reasons a patient may need a pacemaker.
- Have a basic knowledge about how the different types of pacemakers work and what the pacemaker codes represent.
- List the risks associated with having a pacemaker.
- Explain how to exercise a patient with a pacemaker and how the exercise prescription needs to be individualized to that patient based on the type of pacemaker prescribed.

▶ Introduction

Patients can need a pacemaker for many reasons, most often due to a cardiac arrhythmia, atrioventricular (AV) block, sick sinus syndrome, bradycardia, advanced second-degree block, or a hypertrophic dilated cardiomyopathy. Pacemakers can be temporary, such as after heart surgery, or most often permanent to treat a slow heart beat or to improve heart failure symptoms. Patients may report symptoms of fatigue, shortness of breath, fainting, and confusion.

Smaller pacemakers that do not require leads or wires have been developed that can be transplanted directly into the heart. However, many traditional pacemakers with leads are still in use. Pacemakers function by sensing and pacing P and R waves and receiving and processing electrical signals. They may be defined by codes with positions such as DDD, VVI (VDD), VVIR, and DDDR.

- Position 1: chamber or chambers being paced
- Position 2: chamber or chambers being sensed
- Position 3: response for sensing
- Position 4: rate response or rate adaptive pacing

For example, in a DDD pacemaker, the first D represents the area paced; the second D is the area sensed, which is both the atrium and ventricle; and the final D represents what it does (i.e., inhibiting function).

Pacemakers are divided into two main parts: the pulse generator, which is 1 inch or so across and contains the power source and circuitry, and the leads or wires. Sometimes called electrodes, these wires are typically placed in the chamber(s) of the heart. By monitoring your heartbeat and even sensing your body's motion and breathing, pacemakers can speed up heart rate by sending electrical signals to the heart.

There are basically three types of pacemakers. The first type of pacemaker is called a single-chamber pacemaker. This type of pacemaker delivers electrical signals to either the right atria or ventricle of the heart and is typically used to treat symptomatic bradycardia. Next is the dual-chamber pacemaker. Dual-chamber pacemakers carry signals via lead wires to both the right atrium and right ventricle. This type of pacemaker may be used for patients with sinus node dysfunction or AV block. Lastly, biventricular pacemakers are used in patients whose electrical systems are damaged and have congestive heart failure. This type of pacemaker will send electrical signals to both the right ventricle and left ventricle to improve cardiac output.

Risks associated with pacemakers include the following:

- Infection where the pacemaker was implanted
- Allergic reaction to the dye or anesthesia used during the procedure
- Swelling, bruising, or bleeding at the generator site, especially if the patient is taking blood thinners
- Damage to blood vessels or nerves near the pacemaker
- Collapsed lung

A final type of pacemaker is known as an implantable cardio-verter defibrillator, or ICD. These pacemakers are used to treat patients who are at risk for sudden cardiac death with diagnosed sustained ventricular tachycardia or fibrillation. This device basically "shocks" the heart or acts as a cardioverter, and it has preprogrammed activity thresholds set to recognize adverse tachydysrhythmias. Target heart rates should be approximately 10% lower or 10 beats per minute fewer than these preprogrammed activity thresholds to prevent possible discharge of the ICD. Some newer models of ICDs can also function as a pacemaker.

▶ Medications

Typical cardiac medications such as ACE inhibitors, beta-blockers, calcium channel blockers, and vasodilators may be prescribed to patients with pacemakers. Antibiotics also may be necessary at times to treat infections.

▶ Exercise

When exercise-testing patients who are paced with every beat, certain electrocardiogram signs of ischemia, such at ST depression, may not be apparent. For patients with single-chamber pacemakers, such as a VVI, a treadmill or cycle test may not be appropriate, but a 6-minute walk test may provide enough adequate information. A radionuclide test or stress echocardiography also may be performed with good levels of sensitivity. For cardiovascular exercise, a variety of intensity methods may be prescribed depending on the type of pacemaker. For instance, if the patient has a demand pacemaker that only activates when the heart drops below a certain level and is inhibited by the patient's own intrinsic beats, a target heart rate could be appropriate. For patients with fixed-rate pacemakers that stimulate the heart at a predetermined rate, rated perceived exertion (RPE) may be more appropriate.

QUICK-REFERENCE EXERCISE TABLE: PACEMAKERS

Frequency	Intensity	Duration	Modality	Warning Signs
A minimum of 3–5 days per week of aerobic and resistance exercise, if desired	Rated perceived exertion (RPE) of 12–16 on the 6–20 scale	Interval/rest training may be necessary in older or deconditioned patients	Stationary cycle, rower, treadmill, or any other aerobic equipment deemed appropriate	Any swelling or bruising associated with the generator site
Seven days per week may be prescribed provided patient is well-rested and motivated	Target heart rate at an intensity between 50% and 85% of Karvonen for patients with demand-type pacemakers (see Appendix A)	Start with 5–10 minutes at the desired intensity, with rest periods of no more than twice the work minutes, if necessary	For most patients, light hand weights will be appropriate at first; however, more aggressive resistance training may be prescribed depending on age and physical abilities	Any sudden change in energy level; weakness and fatigue
Light hand weights or more aggressive resistance training can be incorporated with each exercise session	Intensity may need to be flexible based on patient's age and changing physical ability and medication (e.g., beta-blockers)	Try to achieve 20–45 minutes of continuous exercise at the prescribed target heart rate or RPE	Other methods of less-supervised exercise, such as swimming and aerobic dance classes, may be appropriate	Rapid weight gain or unusual chest pain

📋 PATIENT QUESTIONS

Are there any types of electrical equipment I should avoid?
Most household electrical appliances, such as microwaves, computers, etc., are safe. However, it is possible that a cell phone may cause interference with your pacemaker. You might want to hold your cell phone on the side of your head opposite from your pacemaker just in case.

Will my pacemaker set off a metal detector?
The metal in your pacemaker may set off a metal detector, but the detector will not interfere with the functioning of your pacemaker.

Can I wear jewelry around my neck?
Yes, jewelry should not interfere with your pacemaker.

What happens if my pacemaker malfunctions?
Only your doctor should put a magnet over your pacemaker; never do it yourself, as it could turn off the pacemaker, depending on the type of pacemaker you have. Your doctor may have done this to test your pacemaker's battery life or to make other adjustments to temporarily reprogram the pacemaker in an asynchronous mode.

What should I do if my implantable cardioverter defibrillator (ICD) fires?
If you receive a shock from your ICD, you will definitely feel it. You should remain calm. If you feel fine, call your doctor's office to let them know. If you are not feeling well and/or receive three or more shocks in a row, call 9-1-1.

Will I always need to have a pacemaker?
After open heart surgery, you may have had a temporary pacemaker. However, in most cases, pacemakers are needed to correct a permanent heart arrhythmia that may have resulted from a previous heart attack or other conduction abnormality.

Notes

Notes

Notes

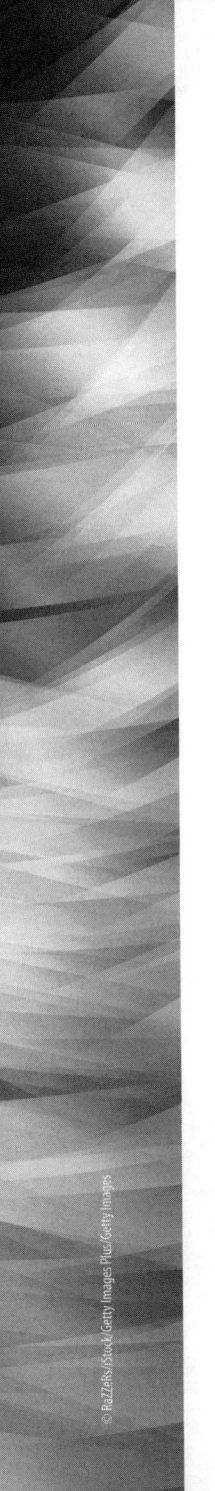

SECTION 2

Other Common Chronic Diseases

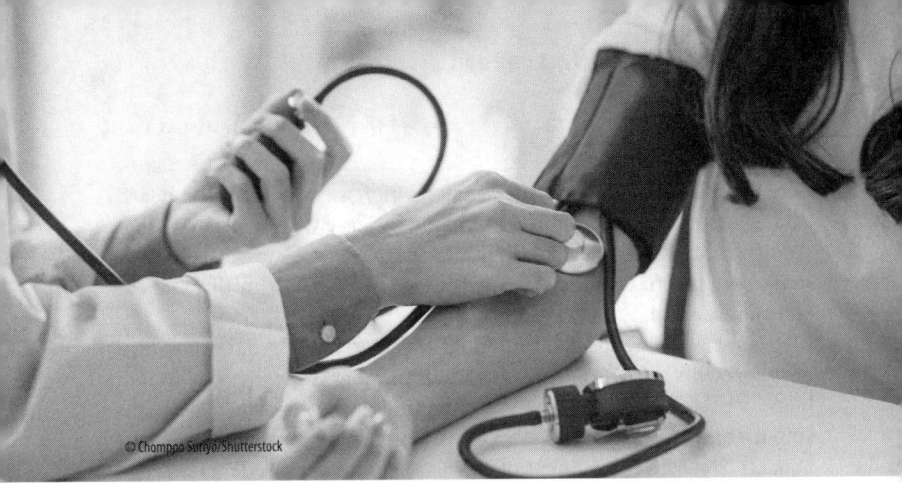

© Chompoo Suriyo/Shutterstock

CHAPTER 8
Hypertension

LEARNING OBJECTIVES

Upon completion of this chapter, the reader will be able to:

- Name the risks for high blood pressure.
- Understand how a normal blood pressure is defined and the most recent risk classifications of blood pressures put forth by the Eighth Joint National Committee.
- Define and explain the difference between the systolic and diastolic blood pressure.
- Identify the blood pressures (i.e., systolic and diastolic) at which exercise should be discontinued.
- Provide a definition of blood pressure using cardiac output and total peripheral resistance.
- Understand how medications prescribed to lower blood pressure may affect exercise.
- List common factors associated with high blood pressure.
- Explain the two types of high blood pressure.

▶ Introduction

High blood pressure, or hypertension, increases the risk for heart disease, stroke, and peripheral vascular disease. Anyone, including young children, can develop high blood pressure. Heart disease and stroke are the first and third leading causes of death in the United States, respectively.

Normal blood pressure is defined as 120/80 mm Hg. The top number represents the systolic pressure. This number is the pressure in the blood vessels when the heart is contracting and should increase with activity or exercise. Individuals with systolic pressures greater than or equal to 200 mm Hg should not exercise, and for most sedentary individuals, exercise should be discontinued if the systolic pressure equals or exceeds 250 mm Hg. The bottom number is called the diastolic pressure. This number represents the pressure in the blood vessels when the heart is relaxing, or in between beats. It should not change or should slightly decrease with activity or exercise, which allows the blood vessels to open or relax so that more blood and oxygen can flow to the working tissues or muscles. If resting diastolic pressures exceed 100–110 mm Hg, exercise is contraindicated. If diastolic pressures equal or exceed 115 mm Hg, activity or exercise should be discontinued.

It is estimated that approximately 50–75 million, or one in three, Americans have high blood pressure. Hypertension may have no symptoms, or patients may experience a pounding in their chest, lightheadedness, dizziness, vision problems, irregular heartbeat, difficulty breathing, and even blood in the urine. Risk factors for hypertension include obesity, excessive alcohol consumption, smoking, and a family history.

Blood pressure (BP) can be defined using the following formula:

BP = cardiac output (CO) × total peripheral resistance (TPR)

Of those who have been diagnosed with hypertensions, only approximately 50% have their blood pressure under control. Common factors associated with hypertension include the following:

- Excessive sodium consumption, greater than 2,400 mg per day
- Blood vessels stiffening and filling with plaque with advancing age
- Smoking
- Poor diets rich in fatty and sugary foods
- Sleep apnea, which causes oxygen levels to decrease when sleeping
- Sedentary lifestyle

Many of the factors listed previously can be controlled. For example, eating fruits and vegetables high in fiber, antioxidants, magnesium, and potassium is associated with improved blood pressure readings. Foods such as blueberries, potatoes, dairy, whole grains such as cereals, beets, and even dark chocolate may reduce the risk for developing hypertension.

Hypertension has two main types: essential (primary or idiopathic) or secondary to another disease. These two types of hypertension account for 90% to 95% of all the cases of high blood pressure. In essential or primary hypertension, the cause is unknown. The majority of hypertension, roughly 90%, falls into this category. Secondary hypertension is caused by another disease such as chronic kidney disease, diabetes, sleep apnea, alcohol addiction, or thyroid disorders.

The classification of blood pressure has recently changed. Since 2003, prehypertension was classified as 120–139 mm Hg systolic and 80–89 mm Hg diastolic. In 2017, the Eighth Joint National Committee reclassified blood pressure. Normal is still less than 120/80 mm Hg. However, they lowered the definition of stage 1 hypertension from 140–159/90–99 mm Hg to 130–139/80–89 mm Hg and added the classification of elevated as 120–129/<80 mm Hg, removing the classification of prehypertension. Stage 2 hypertension was lowered from $\geq$160/100 mm Hg to $\geq$140/90 mm Hg. Finally, a category of hypertensive crisis was added; patients should seek emergency care when blood pressure is higher than 180/120 mm Hg.

It is important to understand that the systolic and diastolic readings should be considered separately when classifying an individual. Only one reading, either the systolic or diastolic, is necessary to be earmarked at the blood pressure classification. The most recent guidelines also emphasize the importance of structured exercise and proper diet to aid in the control of hypertension.

▶ Medications

There are a variety of ways to control hypertension, one of which is antihypertensive medications. It is important to realize that in order to get the maximum benefit from the medicine, exercise and a healthy diet low in refined sugar and fat should be followed. Blood pressure can be controlled either by influencing the central (heart), peripheral (blood vessels) or systemic circulation ($BP = CO \times TPR$). Medications such as beta-blockers act on the heart to reduce blood pressure by blocking beta receptors in the heart that bind catecholamines and increase heart rate and strength of contraction (stroke volume). This results in a drop in resting heart rate of approximately 30 beats per minute and a reduction in stroke volume ($CO = HR \times SV$).

Many of the other medications available to reduce blood pressure work by relaxing or dilating the blood vessels or eliminating fluid build-up in the body. Examples include vasodilators, ACE inhibitors/blockers, calcium channel blockers, and alpha-blockers. These medications may be prescribed alone or in combination. Below are commonly prescribed antihypertensive medications:

- Diuretics
- Beta-blocking and angiotensin-inhibitor drugs
- Angiotensin blockers
- Calcium and alpha-blockers
- Agonists such as alpha-2 receptors
- A combination of alpha- and beta-blockers
- Central agonists
- Vasodilators and peripheral adrenergic inhibitors

▶ Exercise

Obesity and sedentary lifestyle are often strong contributing factors for the development of hypertension. Exercise prescriptions should be developed to address these issues, when necessary, to help reduce blood pressure. For example, by directly tailoring the exercise prescription to optimize caloric expenditure, obesity can be lowered, thus lowering the risk for high blood pressure. Exercise prescriptions that optimize caloric expenditure are typically of lower to moderate aerobic intensity (50% to 70% of VO_2 reserve or heart rate reserve [HRR] using Karvonen's formula) of longer duration and greater frequency. Any percentage of the VO_2 reserve is commensurate with the same percentage of the HRR. Furthermore, small but significant reductions in blood pressure may occur as a result of regular aerobic exercise. This reduction is most often seen in individuals with stage 1 hypertension (130–139/80–89 mm Hg) and lower. Reductions of 5–20 mm Hg per 10 kg of weight loss in both systolic and diastolic readings are possible and may be permanent in patients more than 10% above their ideal body weight.

Patients with hypertension have higher base and peak readings compared to normotensive individuals and may have a delay to baseline blood pressure following exercise. Diastolic readings may even increase during exercise, signifying a possible greater risk for heart attack, stroke, and diabetes. If systolic pressure readings decrease during exercise by 20 mm Hg or more, this could be the result of a weakening heart or excessive vasodilation; exercise should be discontinued and the patient evaluated.

QUICK-REFERENCE EXERCISE TABLE: HYPERTENSION

Frequency	Intensity	Duration	Modality	Warning Signs
A minimum of 3–5 days per week of aerobic and resistance exercise, if desired	Rated perceived exertion (RPE) of 12–16 on the 6–20 scale	Interval/rest training may be necessary in older or deconditioned patients	Stationary cycle, rower, treadmill, or any other aerobic equipment deemed appropriate	Any rapid increases or decreases in blood pressure
Seven days per week may be prescribed, provided patient is well-rested and motivated	Target heart rate at an intensity between 50% and 70% of the VO_2 reserve (see Appendix A)	Start with 5–10 minutes at the desired intensity, with rest periods of no more than twice the work minutes, if necessary	For most patients, light hand weights will be appropriate at first; however, more aggressive resistance training may be prescribed depending on age and physical abilities	Any sudden change in energy level; weakness and fatigue
Light hand weights or more aggressive resistance training can be incorporated with each exercise session	Intensity may need to be flexible based on patient's age and changing physical ability and medication (e.g., beta-blockers)	Try to achieve 20–45 minutes of continuous exercise at the prescribed target heart rate or RPE	Other methods of less-supervised exercise, such as swimming and aerobic dance classes, may be appropriate	Rapid weight gain or unusual chest pain

📋 PATIENT QUESTIONS

I feel fine, yet my doctor tells me I have high blood pressure. How did I get this condition?
The causes of high blood pressure can be multifaceted. For example, age, excessive sodium intake, smoking, diets rich in fat and refined sugar, and lack of a structured exercise program can all contribute to high blood pressure.

I feel the same whether I take my high blood pressure medicine or not. What happens if I forget to take my medicine or just stop?
Hypertension is sometimes called the silent killer. You may not feel any different on or off your medicine, but you may be damaging your heart and blood vessels and you may be at risk for other chronic conditions associated with high blood pressure, such as stroke. If you forget to take your medicine, check with your doctor, but he or she will probably just tell you to resume the medication on schedule the next day.

Will my blood pressure affect my exercise prescription?
It may, as some medications used to treat high blood pressure may lower your heart rate, and if you are exercising by a prescribed target heart rate and your doctor has changed your blood pressure medicine, or the time of day you are taking it, make the healthcare provider who is supervising your exercise aware of this change, as your target heart rate may need to be adjusted. Also, longer, supervised cooldowns may need to be put in place for you, so let your healthcare provider know if you are experiencing any dizziness immediately after exercise.

Why does my healthcare provider advise me to be cautious when taking extended hot showers or baths following exercise?
Some blood pressure medications can relax your blood vessels. This also occurs during exercise and when you are in a hot environment, such as a shower or tub. You may be more likely to get dizzy during these times and should be aware of that and take precautions.

Do my blood pressure medications have any side effects?
Side effects may vary depending on the type of medication you are taking and how your body reacts to the medication. Commonly reported side effects include cough; diarrhea or constipation; lightheadedness; impotency; feeling nervous, weak, tired, or drowsy; headaches; and nausea or vomiting.

Can my high blood pressure cause heart disease? I feel fine and do not have chest pain.
Over time, if your high blood pressure goes untreated or is not diagnosed, it can damage your heart, causing your heart to enlarge. It can also contribute to atherosclerosis or blocked arteries in your body.

Notes

Notes

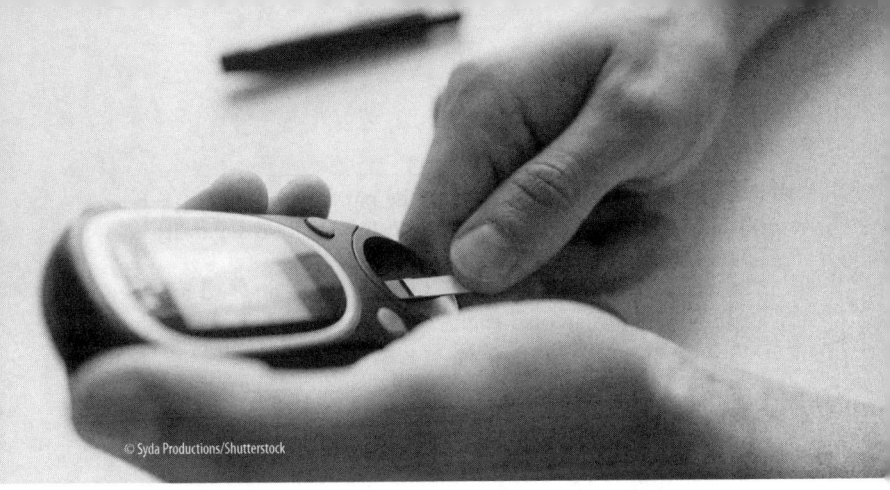

© Syda Productions/Shutterstock

CHAPTER 9
Diabetes

LEARNING OBJECTIVES

Upon completion of this chapter, the reader will be able to:

- Know the history of diabetes.
- List fasting blood glucose levels that represent normal, prediabetes, and diabetes.
- Understand how diabetes is diagnosed and the different tests that can be performed.
- Explain how the glycated hemoglobin test, or HbA1c, is used to evaluate diabetes.
- List risk factors for diabetes.
- Define the three types of diabetes.
- List risk factors associated with diabetes.
- List symptoms associated with diabetes.
- Know when blood sugar levels should be monitored during exercise and at what levels exercise is contraindicated.
- Explain how low blood sugar levels can be corrected prior to, during, and following exercise.
- Know the signs of hypoglycemia.
- Know optimal blood sugar levels for exercise.

▶ **Introduction**

Diabetes is a chronic disease in which the pancreas eventually is no longer able to secrete sufficient insulin to lower blood sugar. It can affect people of any age.

The term *diabetes* can be traced back to 250 BC, and awareness of the disease was noted even earlier, in 400 BC; however, the term did not appear in medical textbooks until around 1425. The full name, *diabetes mellitus,* is Greek for "to siphon or pass through" (referring to excessive urination) and "honey or sweet" (referring to the levels of glucose in the urine). Early diagnosis was performed by tasting the urine of patients, and Early Greek physicians recommended exercise such as horseback riding with the assumption that it would decrease the urge to urinate. The role of the pancreas in insulin production was not discovered until 1889, and it was not until 1921 that insulin was used to treat diabetes in animals. Approximately 350 million people have diabetes worldwide, with 30 million of those cases in the United States, of which approximately 25% are undiagnosed.

The level of glucose (sugar) in blood is measured to diagnosis diabetes. Fasting blood glucose levels greater that 125 mg/dL on two separate occasions and/or a random blood sugar level of 200 mg/dL or higher means the patient has diabetes. Fasting blood sugar levels of 100–125 mg/dL could indicate prediabetes, which is becoming common in obese children. The glycated hemoglobin test, or HbA1c, measures the percentage of blood sugar that attaches to hemoglobin and can be performed to measure the average blood sugar level over the past 2–3 months. An A1c of 6.5% or higher on two separate occasions indicates diabetes; levels of 5.7% to 6.4% indicate prediabetes, while less than 5.7% is considered normal. Blood sugar levels between 160 mg/dL and 180 mg/dL results in a "dumping" of glucose into the urine.

Risk factors for diabetes include the following:

- Family history
- Aging
- Physical inactivity
- Unhealthy diet
- Overweight/obesity
- Smoking
- High blood pressure
- Elevated glucose

Complications of uncontrolled diabetes may result in damage to small blood vessels, which can result in the following:

- Nephropathy (kidney damage)
- Retinopathy (eye damage)
- Heart disease and stroke
- Neuropathies (nerve damage resulting in silent ischemia, or lack of feeling chest pain)
- Foot sores

Diabetes can be broken down into three major types: type I, type II, and gestational diabetes. Only 5% to 10% of patients have type I diabetes, also known as juvenile-onset diabetes. It is believed to be an autoimmune condition affecting the pancreas, where the body's defense mechanisms destroy the pancreatic cells that produce insulin, resulting in little if any insulin production. The lack of insulin results in high blood glucose, muscle breakdown, and ketosis or fat burning. Signs or symptoms of diabetic ketosis are nausea; vomiting; abdominal pain; sweet, fruity breath; and weight loss. This can be a life-threatening condition if elevated toxic acids such as ketones are present in the bloodstream. Many preteens or elementary-aged children diagnosed with type I diabetes are thin and prone to ketosis. Patients with type I diabetes need to take insulin injections to survive. Researchers are not always exactly sure about the cause of type I diabetes, but it is believed that heredity, viral infections, and exposure to harmful environmental factors may play a role.

In type II diabetes, insulin levels can be elevated, reduced, or somewhat normal. In most cases, insulin levels rise as obesity increases, resulting in greater and greater insulin resistance. Eventually, the pancreas "tires," the beta cells fatigue in the pancreas, and it can no longer produce insulin. Approximately 90% of type II diabetics are older and obese with a family history of diabetes. However, it has been reported recently by the Centers for Disease Control and Prevention that more than 5,000 new cases are diagnosed in the United States each year among those younger than 20 years of age! Oral medications may be prescribed to maintain insulin output. Some of these oral medications may stimulate the pancreas to secrete insulin; others may inhibit the production and release of glucose from the liver; and, finally, some may block the stomach from breaking down carbohydrates and may make tissues more sensitive to insulin. However, if diet, exercise, and weight loss are not achieved, these oral drugs may no longer be effective, and the patient may need to be put on insulin injections permanently. Pancreatic transplantation and bariatric surgery are much more invasive options. Transplantation is usually performed in type I diabetics. Bariatric surgery may be performed to help control blood sugar levels in patients with body mass index greater than 35.

Symptoms for both type I and type II diabetes include the following:

- Weight loss
- Blurred vision
- Tiredness
- Excessive thirst and urination
- Hunger
- Delayed wound healing
- Numbness in hands and feet

The third type of diabetes is known as gestational diabetes, and it occurs in 2% to 10% of pregnancies in the United States. The exact cause of gestational diabetes is not known for sure; however, it is believed that hormones that affect the placenta, such as human placental lactogen, increase insulin resistance. Screening for gestational diabetes includes the monitoring and measuring of blood sugar levels between weeks 24 and 28 of pregnancy. Gestational diabetes usually resolves following delivery; however, individuals have a 50% chance of developing diabetes later in life. Risk factors for gestational diabetes include the following:

- Obesity prior to and during pregnancy
- Having gestational diabetes during a past pregnancy
- A parent, sibling, or child with diabetes
- Previous delivery of large birth weight infants over 9 pounds
- Complications during pregnancy
- Older than 25 years
- Expecting multiple births
- Unexplained miscarriage or stillbirth
- Have been prescribed glucocorticoids

▶ Medications

Diabetes is managed by a variety of medications, such as insulin injections, oral agents, antihypertensives, and lipid-lowering agents designed to control blood sugar levels and reduce the associated risk for heart disease. Categories of medications prescribed to treat type II diabetes are as follows:

- Alpha-glucosidase inhibitors aid in carbohydrate digestion.
- Biguanides such as metformin decrease the liver's production of glucose and increase the body's absorption while making one more sensitive to insulin.

- Dopamine agonists may decrease insulin resistance.
- DPP-4 inhibitors reduce blood sugar.
- Glucagon-like peptides increase B-cell growth in the pancreas.
- Meglitinides help the body to release insulin.
- Sodium glucose transporter 2 inhibitors help the kidney to eliminate glucose via the urine.
- Sulfonylureas stimulate the pancreas to secrete more insulin.
- Thiazolidinediones decrease glucose in the liver and help fat cells use insulin better.

The treatment for type I diabetes, where the pancreas produces little if any insulin, usually requires insulin. Insulin is typically administered by injection; however, it also can be delivered by an insulin pump. Insulin pumps are approximately the size of a deck of cards and are designed to deliver insulin via a catheter inserted under the skin. There also is a wireless pump option that involves a pod and tiny catheter inserted under the skin. A wireless device can then be used to program the pod. Pumps are designed to dispense rapid-acting insulin automatically and are preprogrammed to deliver the insulin based on carbohydrate intake. Insulin injections may contain short-acting (regular) insulin, rapid-acting insulin, intermediate-acting insulin, and long-acting insulin.

A final type of treatment for diabetes is called an artificial pancreas. This device continuously monitors blood glucose every few minutes, linked to an insulin pump. It can then automatically deliver the correct amount of insulin when needed.

Blood sugar levels usually need to be checked at least four times per day. The American Diabetes Association recommends checking blood sugar levels before bed, meals, and snacks and prior to driving. Blood sugar can be tested using a variety of methods or tools. If the patient does not have an insulin pump monitoring his or her blood glucose, a finger prick with a small lancet may be done to produce a drop of blood, which can then be placed on a test strip and analyzed. Even smart phones are now being used to monitor blood glucose levels via sensors under the skin that measure intestinal glucose; these are known as continuous glucose monitors and help prevent frequent finger pricks. Noninvasive infrared glucose monitoring using mid-infrared absorption spectroscopy to measure blood glucose is becoming more popular.

▶ Exercise

Blood sugar should be monitored prior, during, and following exercise when patients have been sedentary or are unfamiliar with how exercise may affect their blood sugar. If blood sugar levels are greater than 250–300 mg/dL, exercise should be postponed, as blood sugar levels this elevated could increase when the muscles release glucose during exercise. The patient should contact his or her physician, who may adjust the insulin medication. If blood glucose levels are between 80 and 100 mg/dL, 15–30 g of carbohydrate should be ingested before, during, or after vigorous long-term exercise and blood sugar levels retested. If blood sugar levels are less than 70 mg/dL, exercise should be postponed to prevent possible hypoglycemia. Symptoms of hypoglycemia are as follows:

- Dizziness
- Extreme hunger
- Headache and confusion
- Sweating and shaking
- Blurred vision

Blood sugar levels of 100–250 mg/dL are optimal for exercise.

Other factors to consider prior, during, and after exercise are as follows:

- Type and timing of medications
- The previous meal
- Intensity, duration. and type of exercise
- Any symptoms that may warrant checking blood glucose
- Avoid exercise during peak insulin times to decrease the likelihood of hypoglycemia
- Caution when exercising in extreme heat

The preferred site for insulin injection is the abdomen; however, the thigh and back of the arm also may be used. Injecting insulin into muscle groups that will be actively used during exercise should be avoided as much as possible to prevent increased absorption of insulin due to increased circulation at the injection site.

People with diabetes run a greater risk for heart disease and stroke because, over time, high blood glucose can damage the nerves and blood vessels that control the heart. Therefore, a regular exercise program can improve cardiovascular health, promote weight loss in obese patients, improve musculoskeletal strength, and reduce stress.

QUICK-REFERENCE EXERCISE TABLE: DIABETES

Frequency	Intensity	Duration	Modality	Warning Signs
A minimum of 3–5 days per week of aerobic and resistance exercise, if desired	Rated perceived exertion (RPE) of 12–16 on the 6–20 scale	Interval/rest training may be necessary in older or deconditioned patients	Stationary cycle, rower, treadmill, or any other aerobic equipment deemed appropriate	Signs of hypoglycemia
Seven days per week may be prescribed provided patient is well-rested and motivated or has type II diabetes and is obese	Target heart rate at an intensity between 50% and 70% of Karvonen or the VO_2 reserve (see Appendix A)	Start with 5–10 minutes at the desired intensity, with rest periods of no more than twice the work minutes, if necessary	For most patients, light hand weights will be appropriate at first; however, more aggressive resistance training may be prescribed depending on age and physical abilities	Any sudden change in energy level; weakness and fatigue; or sudden increase or decrease in blood pressure
Light hand weights or more aggressive resistance training can be incorporated with each exercise session	Intensity may need to be flexible based on patient's age and changing physical ability and medication (e.g., beta-blockers)	Try to achieve 20–60 minutes of continuous exercise at the prescribed target heart rate or RPE. For patients needing to lose weight, prescribe exercise at the low end of the intensity window and increase the frequency and duration to maximize caloric expenditure.	Other methods of less-supervised exercise, such as swimming and aerobic dance classes, may be appropriate	Rapid changes in weight or unusual chest pain

📋 PATIENT QUESTIONS

Will I have diabetes all my life?
If you are told you have type I diabetes, then yes. If you are a type II diabetic, you are most likely will have diabetes for the rest of your life if you are using injectable insulin. If you are on antidiabetic pills and can reduce your risk factors for diabetes, such as obesity, you may not have to inject insulin.

Does having diabetes put me at risk for other medical problems?
Yes, you may be at a greater risk for heart disease, stroke, and other organ problems.

How often should I test my blood sugar?
Usually the frequency depends on which type of diabetes you have and if you have a continuous glucose monitoring device. You doctor may recommend you check your blood sugar as many as 10 times per day if you have type I diabetes; if you have type II diabetes, check at least every day, preferably a couple of hours before and after meals. You may not have to check your blood sugar if you have prediabetes.

How often should I check my blood sugar when I am exercising?
If you have never exercised or are changing the intensity, duration, and/or frequency of your exercise, you might consider checking your blood sugar before, during, and after exercise or if you feel any signs of hypoglycemia.

Should I eat any special kinds of foods to manage my diabetes?
Nothing should be completely off-limits, but you should avoid or limit foods high in refined simple sugars, such as sodas and sugary cereals; processed grains like white rice, white bread, and flour; and foods high in trans fats. Good choices are whole grains like brown rice, oatmeal, sweet potatoes, and other foods that contain little or no added sugar. Load up on fresh fruits and vegetables!

Why do I have diabetes?
Many factors can contribute to diabetes, such as diet, obesity, viral infections, and even heredity. Some of the risk factors for diabetes are controllable. Talk to your healthcare provider and know which type of diabetes you have, what you can do to prevent it from getting worse, and the best way to control your diabetes.

Notes

Notes

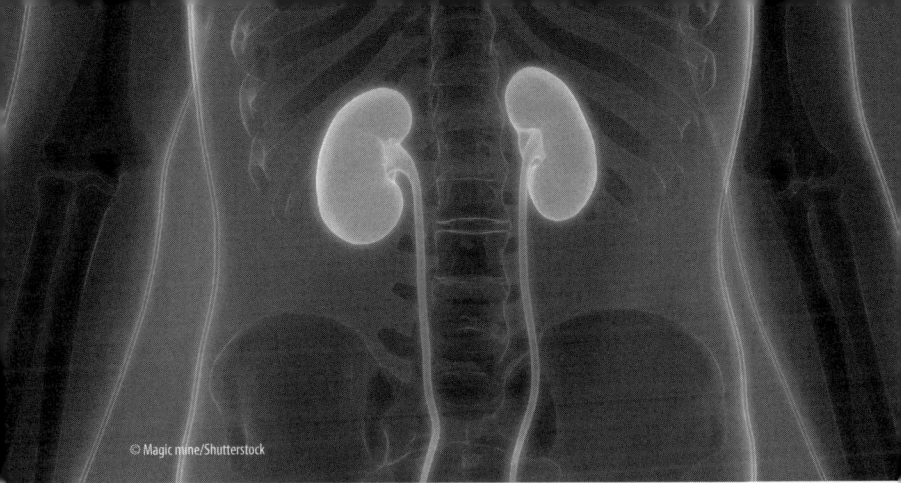

CHAPTER 10
Kidney Disease

▶ Introduction

Kidney disease can occur over months or years. Seventy percent of kidney failure in the United States is associated with a disease or condition, such as type II diabetes or hypertension, that impairs kidney function. Many symptoms associated with kidney failure are nonspecific and can be common to other conditions; for example, nausea, shortness of breath, sleep problems, muscle twitches, swelling of the ankles, and chest pain are just a few of the commonly reported symptoms of kidney failure.

Family history, premature birth, trauma or an accident, and advancing age all can be risk factors for kidney disease. Other causes of or risk factors for kidney failure are as follows:

- Diseases that attack the blood vessels and nephrons in the kidneys
- Type I diabetes
- Polycystic diseases (fluid-filled bubbles in the kidneys)
- Tumors or cancers
- Lupus
- Use of nonsteroidal anti-inflammatory drugs (NSAIDS) such as ibuprofen, naproxen, and acetaminophen
- Birth defects and unknown causes
- African American, Native American, or Asian American ethnicity

Kidney failure can be treated, but not cured, and is most commonly seen in ages 40 to 60 years. The main role of the kidneys is to keep the body's chemistry in check. It does this by making urine to get rid of wastes. Other roles associated with the kidneys include the following:

- Balance minerals
- Blood pressure control
- Manufacture of red blood cells (erythropoietin)
- Maintenance of bone health
- Normalize Ph levels

Patients diagnosed with kidney failure or on dialysis can experience many consequences that can affect their daily activities. A condition known as secondary hyperparathyroidism involves excessive secretion of parathyroid hormone, which results in low blood calcium and bone and joint pain and deformation. Another associated problem is called renal osteodystrophy. It occurs when the kidneys fail to maintain proper levels of calcium and phosphorous, causing bone disease and stunted growth in children. Peripheral nerves connecting the brain and spinal cord can become damaged or diseased, which can impair muscle movement and prevent normal sensation in the arms and legs, causing pain. Patients also may have elevations in cholesterol and triglycerides, accelerating the chance of atherosclerosis and heart disease.

▶ **Medications**

Kidney disease and failure can be managed in several ways. Many patients with kidney disease do not make enough of the hormone called erythropoietin, resulting in anemia. A medication called erythropoiesis, a stimulating agent, may be prescribed. Phosphate and potassium binders also may be prescribed to help get rid of high levels of these compounds in the blood. Supplements containing vitamin D, calcium, and iron also may be needed.

Chronic kidney failure and end-stage renal disease may result in the need for dialysis and/or kidney transplant. There are two types of dialysis: hemodialysis and peritoneal dialysis. Hemodialysis involves a machine, usually located in a dialysis center, that filters and cleans the blood. This is the most common treatment for kidney failure. Peritoneal dialysis uses the lining of the stomach as a filter to clean the blood. It involves a tube or catheter inserted into the stomach that instills hypertonic cleansing fluid to remove waste products from the blood. This type of dialysis can be done almost anywhere. Lastly, a kidney transplant may be necessary for survival of the patient. Most kidney transplants are performed on patients who are currently on dialysis and have no kidney function or are considered pre-emptive with some kidney functionality. Donors can be hard to find, coupled with a lack of access to transplant centers and low rates of referrals for patients in lower socioeconomic levels.

▶ **Exercise**

Prescribing exercise for patients with kidney disease or in kidney failure can be a challenge, especially if they are on dialysis. Patients typically have low MET levels just above activities of daily living (ADLs) around 5.7 METs. Furthermore, they may exhibit a blunted heart rate response, early fatigue, anemia, and muscle and joint pain. Following 3 months of training, it is not uncommon for patients to demonstrate a 20% to 25% increase in exercise capacity. In patients receiving some form of dialysis, exercise timing is important. For those patients who need to have an exercise test, it is recommended that the test be performed on nondialysis days. Exercise training is best done during dialysis, preferably with a stationary cycle. Exercise before dialysis or immediately after dialysis is not recommended because blood chemistries may be poor before dialysis and patients are typically fatigued following dialysis.

QUICK-REFERENCE EXERCISE TABLE: KIDNEY DISEASE

Frequency	Intensity	Duration	Modality	Warning Signs
Three times per week or during dialysis treatments	Rated perceived exertion (RPE) of 10–14 on the 6–20 scale	Interval/rest training may be necessary in deconditioned patients	Stationary cycle is the recommended modality	Report any changes in phosphate, calcium, or potassium levels
Immediately following dialysis, the patient may be fatigued	Target heart rate intensities are not appropriate	Start with 5–10 minutes at the desired intensity, with rest periods of no more than twice the work minutes, if necessary	Other modalities can be applied on a case-by-case basis	Any sudden change in energy level, weakness, fatigue, nausea, or blood pressure changes
Predialysis, the patient's blood chemistries may not be optimal	Patients may have a blunted heart rate response to exercise	Try to achieve 20–60 minutes of continuous exercise at the prescribed RPE	Other methods of less-supervised exercise, such as swimming and aerobic dance classes, may be appropriate	Rapid changes in weight or unusual chest pain and muscle cramps

📋 PATIENT QUESTIONS

My doctor has told me that I have chronic kidney disease. Will I have to have dialysis?
The early stages of chronic kidney disease can last for many years. If your kidneys fail and you are on dialysis waiting for a new kidney, a kidney transplant will be needed to keep you alive.

What types of dialysis options are there?
Basically, there are two options: peritoneal dialysis and hemodialysis. Peritoneal dialysis may be done at home with a tube surgically inserted in your abdomen. Hemodialysis is usually done at a center, but can take place at home as well.

When will I know when it's time for dialysis?
Your doctor will be monitoring your kidneys and let you know in plenty of time to prepare you. Usually, dialysis is recommended when your kidney function drops to 15% or less. If you have symptoms of shortness of breath, muscle cramps, fatigue, nausea, or vomiting, let your doctor know immediately.

Will insurance cover dialysis?
If you have private insurance, you should be covered. If you are on state- or federally funded program, such as Medicare or Medicaid, you may be covered up to a minimum of 80%.

How long can I stay on dialysis, and will I eventually need a kidney transplant?
Some people have had dialysis for 30 or more years without getting a transplant. It will depend on how well you take care of yourself and taking an active role in your health care.

Why did I get kidney disease?
There is a good chance that your kidney failure was associated with a disease or condition, such as type II diabetes or hypertension, that impaired your kidney function.

Notes

Notes

_____
_____
_____
_____
_____
_____
_____
_____
_____
_____
_____
_____
_____
_____
_____
_____
_____
_____
_____
_____
_____
_____
_____
_____
_____

Notes

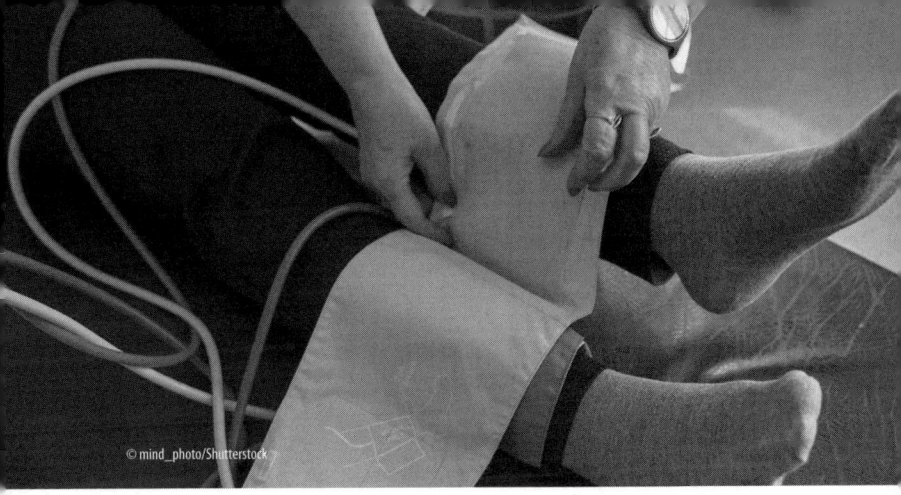

© mind_photo/Shutterstock

CHAPTER 11

Peripheral Arterial Disease

▶ **Introduction**

Peripheral arterial disease (PAD), sometimes called peripheral vascular disease, is a circulatory problem that involves narrowed arteries (i.e., claudication), most commonly the legs but also in the head, stomach, and arms. As many as eight million people in the United States are have PAD and are at an increased risk for heart disease. It is commonly diagnosed in patients who are older than 40 years. Risk factors for PAD include hypertension, elevated cholesterol, smoking, family history of heart disease, and diabetes.

Patients diagnosed with PAD often have intermittent claudication, resulting in muscle pain, cramping, and numbness in the calf and other leg muscles. PAD symptoms' severity may be graded on a 0–3 scale, with 0 meaning asymptomatic and 3 meaning major or minor tissue loss from the foot. Other symptoms include the following:

- Slow healing of foot and/or toe sores
- Gangrene
- Cold feet
- Poor nail growth
- Poor hair growth on the legs
- Impotence in men with diabetes

Arteries commonly affected in the lower limbs are the iliac, femoral, popliteal, dorsalis pedis, and tibial arteries. There are close to three million new reported cases of PAD each year; if it goes untreated, the kidneys may begin to fail and, in severe instances, leg amputation and heart attacks may result.

The evaluation of PAD can occur in several ways. A standard test done to evaluate the existence of PAD is known as the Strandness test, developed by Dr. Eugene Strandness, known as the father of the vascular laboratory. The Strandness test involves having the patient walk on a treadmill slowly at 2 mph with the grade increased by 2% every 2 minutes until the patient can no longer continue, or the patient may begin at 2 mph and a 12% grade with a set walking time of 5 minutes. Maximal walking time and claudication pain times are recorded. Following the treadmill test, ankle-brachial index, or ABI, measurements can be performed to measure the severity of PAD. This test involves comparing the systolic blood pressure in the leg or ankle (dorsalis pedis artery) to the systolic blood pressure in the arm (brachial artery) using a doppler sphygmomanometer (ankle pressure/arm pressure). An ABI score of less than <1.0 is abnormal. This score also can be compared to a resting ABI to determine the degree of claudication resulting from the exercise test. Other diagnostic tests may include a doppler ultrasound to evaluate blood flow, angiography involving a catheter, or angiography using imaging techniques such as magnetic resonance angiography and computerized tomography angiography. Finally, blood tests should be done to measure risk factors for artery disease, such as lipids and cholesterol.

▶ Medications

The treatment for PAD has two main goals. The first is to manage symptoms of leg pain and improve walking distance, and the second is to slow the progression of atherosclerosis, reducing the chance of worsening symptoms and decreasing the risk for heart attacks and strokes. To achieve these goals, exercise, smoking cessation, lifestyle changes, and medications should all be discussed. In some instances, more invasive treatment may be needed, such as angioplasty or bypass surgery.

Follows is a list of medications that may be prescribed to manage PAD:

- Cholesterol-lowering medications (statins). The goal being to reduce the low-density lipoproteins (so-called bad cholesterol) to less than 100 mg/dL.
- Hypertensive medications to reduce blood pressure to 130/80 mm Hg or less.
- Blood thinners to reduce the chance of blood clots.
- Medications to increase blood flow to the legs, such as cilostazol and pentoxifylline.

Patients with PAD should avoid cold medications containing pseudoephedrine because they may constrict blood vessels and worsen symptoms. In some patients taking beta-blockers, a decrease in claudication time has been reported. Patient with PAD who are also diabetic should monitor and control their diabetes and blood sugar; they should also pay attention to proper foot care.

▶ Exercise

As discussed earlier, a Strandness treadmill test and/or ABI measurements may be done to evaluate maximal walking and claudication times, indicating the severity of PAD. However, patients with PAD will likely have accompanying coronary artery disease, and a doctor may often prescribe an exercise test to rule out coronary artery disease or possibly to reevaluate maximal walking and claudication pain times.

If the goal is to rule out coronary artery disease, the best modality to use is an electronically braked stationary cycle ergometer; testing on a treadmill may fatigue the leg muscles early and claudication may limit the duration of the test. Therefore, the patient may not achieve an adequate heart rate and blood pressure to rule out coronary artery disease on the treadmill.

The favored modality to improve maximal walking time in the PAD patient is the treadmill. Interval training on the treadmill likely will need to be prescribed, along with active rest exercise periods to improve cardiovascular health. Active rest exercise involves having the patient continue to exercise on another modality until the leg pain subsides, as opposed to sitting in a chair and resting. When claudication pain reaches 3 or 4 on the claudication pain scale (the maximum is 4) on the treadmill, or the patient is at the maximal walking time and can no longer continue, active rest exercise should be initiated. It may be done on the arm ergometer, seated rowing machine, or the stationary cycle ergometer, as these are recommended modalities for leg pain recovery and likely available in any cardiac rehabilitation center. The purpose of active rest exercise is to improve cardiovascular conditioning, and it should be performed until the leg pain subsides enough to resume exercise on the treadmill. Ideally, the active rest exercise periods should decrease over time and the maximal walking time on the treadmill should increase. This will encourage improvements in collateral circulation; reduce blood viscosity; and improve aerobic capacity, walking efficiency, and pain tolerance.

QUICK-REFERENCE EXERCISE TABLE: PERIPHERAL ARTERIAL DISEASE

Frequency	Intensity	Duration	Modality	Warning Signs
Three to seven times per week as recovery tolerates	Walking exercise to 3 or 4 on the claudication pain scale, where 4 is the maximum	Interval/rest training may be necessary for most patients	Treadmill is the recommended modality to improve walking distance and time	Report any chest pain immediately to the healthcare professional
Walking exercise may be performed daily to maximize continuous walking time	Target heart rate intensities may not be appropriate if maximal walking times limit the achievement of a target heart rate	Walking should be performed until the patient can no longer continue	Other modalities such as stationary cycles, arm ergometers, and even rowers can be applied during the active rest exercise periods	Any sudden change in energy level or weakness, fatigue, nausea or blood pressure changes
Walking exercise can be performed at home on off days	Target heart rates can be prescribed once walking time reaches a minimum of 20 continuous minutes	Once the patient can no longer continue to walk, an active rest exercise modality should be prescribed until the patient can resume activity on the treadmill. Try to achieve a minimum of 20 minutes of continuous walking.	Other methods of less-supervised exercise such as swimming, aerobic dance classes, and resistance training may be appropriate once maximal walking times have exceeded 20 minutes	Rapid changes in weight

📝 PATIENT QUESTIONS

Why did I get peripheral arterial disease?
If you smoked, have high blood pressure and/or diabetes, are sedentary, and/or have elevated cholesterol, these are all factors that contribute to PAD.

Am I at a risk for other diseases?
Yes, you may be at a greater risk for coronary heart disease and stroke.

Is my disease temporary or permanent?
Peripheral arterial disease is total body disease affecting your arteries, and it results in the blockage or narrowing of your arteries. It can occur in many areas of your body. It can be controlled, but you will have to work on lowering the risk factors for PAD and exercise regularly.

Why did my doctor tell me to pay attention to my feet?
Peripheral arterial disease results in poor circulation to your muscles. If injuries or sores occur on your lower legs and feet, this can put you at risk for poor healing and infection.

Why did my doctor recommend I sleep with my head and chest raised?
Keeping your legs below the level of your heart may increase circulation and reduce pain. You should also avoid cold temperatures as much as possible to reduce pain.

What should I do when I am exercising or walking and feel pain in my calves?
Try to exercise or walk as long as you can tolerate the pain. This may help to eventually improve the circulation in your legs. If you feel chest pain, stop immediately and seek medical attention.

Notes

Notes

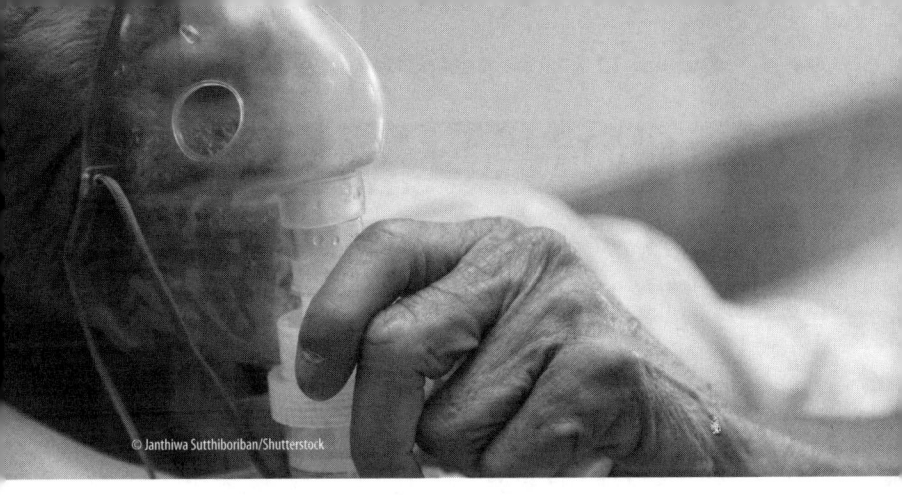

CHAPTER 12

Chronic Obstructive Pulmonary Disease (COPD)

LEARNING OBJECTIVES

Upon completion of this chapter, the reader will be able to:

- Explain the differences between chronic bronchitis, asthma, and emphysema.
- Identify the differences between obstructive and restrictive lung diseases.
- Understand how chronic obstructive pulmonary disease (COPD) is diagnosed and how testing is performed.
- Name factors other than smoking that can result in damage to the alveoli in the lungs.

(continues)

LEARNING OBJECTIVES   *(continued)*

- Understand the importance of alpha$_1$-antitrypsin deficiencies in lung damage.
- Define the terms "Blue Bloaters" and "Pink Puffers."
- Describe the technique of pursed-lip breathing and how it can be taught to improve breathing.
- List things that can trigger asthmatic attacks.
- Understand how medications used to treat COPD can be used before, during, and after exercise.
- List the aerobic benefits of exercise for COPD patients.
- Explain hypoxia and how it is associated with oxygen saturation (SaO$_2$).
- Understand how to monitor SaO$_2$ and identify normal levels.
- Know what a Spirotiger-type device is and how it can be used to strengthen ventilatory muscles.
- Know how to use the dyspnea scale when prescribing and monitoring exercise.

▶ Introduction

Under the umbrella of chronic obstructive pulmonary disease (COPD) are emphysema, chronic bronchitis, and sometimes asthma. COPD worsens over time, making it increasingly difficult to breathe. The diagnosis of COPD should be confirmed by having a pulmonary function test or spirometry. This test involves the patient blowing air into a tube connected to a device called a spirometer, and the amount and speed of air that comes out of the lungs are measured. Normal spirometry values can vary based on the patient's size, age, and gender, but they are usually considered normal when the forced expiratory volume (FEV$_1$), the amount of air exhaled in 1 second after taking a deep breath, is 80% to 120% of the predicted value. Another measurement involves the ratio of the forced vital capacity (FVC) to the FEV$_1$. A ratio of 0.7 or less is considered normal.

COPD is a chronic inflammation of the lungs that results in obstructed air flow. Most patients experience a cough; difficulty breathing; excessive mucus or sputum production, especially in the morning; and wheezing. Smoking is one of the most common causes of COPD. Patients with COPD have a greater risk for heart disease, lung cancer, and other diseases. The most common components COPD are emphysema and chronic bronchitis.

Emphysema is a condition where the alveoli are permanently damaged. The alveoli are tiny, balloon-shaped air sacs that, when healthy, resemble a cluster of grapes. Their purpose in the lungs is to exchange oxygen and carbon dioxide into and out of the bloodstream. They are located at the distal end of the respiratory tree and throughout the lungs. It has been estimated that the surface of the healthy alveoli could span the area of a tennis court, making them valuable structures in the exchange of oxygen and carbon dioxide. When alveoli become damaged, their surface area is permanently reduced, and they resemble more of a solid, round structure or are "orange-like" in appearance. There are a number of factors other than smoking that can cause the alveoli to become inflamed and damaged, which include the following:

- Pneumonia
- Tuberculosis
- Lung cancers
- Acute respiratory distress syndrome (ARDS), typically seen in critically ill patients
- Pulmonary edema
- Alpha$_1$-antitrypsin deficiency, a rare, inherited condition that allows harmful enzymes to remain in the lungs, resulting in lung destruction

As air becomes trapped in the alveoli, it causes them to lose their elasticity and makes it difficult to exhale in patients with emphysema; patients often have a hyperinflated or "barrel" chest. Patients with severe emphysema are referred to by an old term known as "pink puffers" because they have trouble oxygenating and may appear thin and catabolic with little or no cough. A technique known as pursed-lip breathing should be applied to help the patient exhale trapped air in the lungs. This technique involves teaching the patient to exhale with closed lips, as though they are about to whistle; this helps to increase the pressure in the chest, slow down the expiration, and expel the carbon dioxide to feel less shortness of breath. This technique has been shown to be very successful when performed properly.

Most patients with COPD have a combination of both emphysema and chronic bronchitis. Chronic bronchitis, or "blue bloaters" (an old term), is a severe long-term condition where the bronchial tubes become inflamed and constricted. These patients are typically overweight, blue in color around the lips and fingertips, and have shortness of breath and a chronic cough. These patients produce excess muus or sputum, causing the airways to become more constricted, resulting in a chronic cough. Patients with chronic bronchitis are typically obese and present with an expectorant cough with wheezing. Some patients may show signs of right-sided heart failure (cor pulmonale) with ankle edema and cyanosis. Environmental pollutants, bacterial infections, and cigarette smoking are but a few of the major factors that may contribute to chronic bronchitis and COPD. These patients also have trouble exhaling; a chest X-ray may be performed to rule out other lung problems. Polycythemia or an abnormally elevated concentration of red blood cells may also be present and, if not treated, can result in blood clots, leading to heart attacks and strokes.

Asthma, also under the umbrella of COPD, is a chronic lung disease that involves inflammation and narrowing of the airways in the lungs. Chest tightness, wheezing, and coughing usually occur at night or in the early morning. Asthma can be triggered by allergies, coughs, environmental pollutants, dust mites, medications, and exercise. Patients with asthma have narrowed airways that swell and produce excessive mucus, resulting in coughing and wheezing. Asthma cannot be cured, but the symptoms can be controlled with medications and avoidance of triggers. Asthma can flare up in certain situations such as exercise, especially in dry, cold climates and in the presence of a variety of allergy triggers. Asthma symptoms can be measured using a peak flow meter to check how well the lungs are working. Flow meters are portable, inexpensive, and can be hand-held. They measure how air leaves the lungs and can show changes in the lungs before they are felt. Patients with emphysema and chronic bronchitis also may benefit using a peak flow meter to help determine any changes in lung function and adjust medications to their specific COPD plan.

The majority of patients with COPD will have an obstructive component to their lung disease, or difficulty exhaling; however, some will also have a restrictive component, or difficulty inhaling. Like COPD, restrictive disease progressively gets worse over time; however, in some cases this disease can be reversed.

Patients with restrictive disease suffer many of the same symptoms as to COPD patients. In restrictive lung disease, the lungs have a difficult time expanding and are "stiff." Conditions that can lead to restrictive lung disease include the following:

- Pulmonary fibrosis, a condition where scar tissue builds up in the lungs
- Sarcoidosis involving masses or lumps in the lungs
- Obesity
- Scoliosis of the spine
- Muscular dystrophy and amyotrophic lateral sclerosis

▶ Medications

There is no cure for COPD. However, medications are available that can help to reduce the inflammation in the lungs and improve breathing. Commonly prescribed medications are bronchodilators, taken in either pill form or by an inhaler. Other medications include the following:

- Short-acting sympathomimetics or bronchodilators may be used for quick relief to open airways. Albuterol is an example of such a medication.
- Corticosteroids reduce inflammation. Prednisone is a commonly prescribed corticosteroid.
- Methylxanthines or theophylline.
- Long-acting bronchodilators to reduce inflammation and improve breathing over a longer period of time.
- Cromolyn sodium, an anti-inflammatory medication used in allergic reactions.
- Leukotriene receptor antagonists to block bronchoconstriction.

▶ Exercise

Exercise by itself cannot reverse COPD or directly improve lung parameters, but aerobic exercise can improve circulation by helping the body to make better use of the oxygen that is supplied to the muscles so the patient can do more activities without becoming short of breath, thus improving quality of life. Patients with COPD usually begin by exercising in a structured program recommended to them by their physician, two days per week (Tuesdays and Thursdays). All patients with COPD should be instructed on how to do pursed-lip breathing to lower the amount of air trapped in the lungs and reduce shortness of breath during exercise. Patients with chronic bronchitis usually perform better in the afternoon once the mucus or sputum has had a chance to clear from the lungs. Further benefits of aerobic exercise for COPD patients include the following:

- Strengthen the heart and circulatory system
- Lower blood pressure
- Improve muscle strength, tone and flexibility
- Strengthen bones
- Reduce body fat
- Relieve stress, anxiety, and depression
- Improve sleep patterns
- Boost self-esteem
- Reduce fear of dyspnea

If possible, the exercise environment should be warm and humid and include a mild warm-up period; cold, dry environments are more likely to result in constriction of the lungs. Before exercising, patients should be coached on the pursed-lip breathing technique discussed earlier. Oxygen saturation levels (SaO_2) also may need to be monitored prior to and during exercise to make sure the patient maintains a SaO_2 level above 88%. If SaO_2 levels fall below 88% and hypoxemia occurs for an extended time, exercise intensity should be reduced and the patient's physician notified to see if supplemental oxygen is needed. If untreated, hypoxemia can result in polycythemia and erythrocytosis, the excessive production of red blood cells. This can lead to an increase in blood viscosity and an increased chance of strokes and heart attacks.

Ventilatory muscles can be strengthened using hand-held devices. One such device is called a Spirotiger. Its application has been used to improve the amount of air that moves in and out of the lungs, or tidal volume (TV), and reduce dyspnea. This device also may be used to access the ventilatory equivalents (V_E). The ventilatory equivalent, or minute volume, is the ratio of ventilation to oxygen intake or carbon dioxide output. It can be expressed as the product of TV and the frequency of breaths per minute. The Spirotiger can be used by both athletes and individuals with lung diseases.

To monitor exercise intensity, a target heart rate may not be appropriate in patients who are limited by the severity of their lung disease. For those individuals, using a subjective dyspnea scale (0–10) is recommended. A dyspnea rating of 3–6, representing between 50% and 85% of the VO_2max, should be prescribed.

QUICK-REFERENCE EXERCISE TABLE: CHRONIC OBSTRUCTIVE PULMONARY DISEASE

Frequency	Intensity	Duration	Modality	Warning Signs
Two to seven times per week as recovery allows	Exercise at 3–6 on the 0–10 dyspnea chart	Interval/rest training may be necessary for most patients	Treadmill is the recommended modality to begin with to evaluate lung parameters and dyspnea	Report any chest pain immediately to the healthcare professional
Exercise may be performed daily to maximize caloric expenditure if the patient is obese, as in chronic bronchitis	Target heart rate intensities may not be appropriate if the patient's exercise is limited by lung parameters	Aerobic exercise should be performed initially	Other modalities such as stationary cycles, arm ergometers, and even rowers can be applied. Resistance training can be prescribed once aerobic exercise reaches a continuous 20 minutes or more	Any sudden change in energy level, weakness, fatigue, nausea, or blood pressure changes
Exercise can be performed at home on off days	Target heart rates at 50% to 70% of Karvonen or heart rate reserve (HRR) can be prescribed once the exercise intensity and duration allows	The goal for aerobic exercise duration should be a continuous 20–60 minutes	Other methods of less-supervised exercise, such as swimming, aerobic dance classes, or resistance training may be appropriate once maximal aerobic times have exceeded 20 minutes	Rapid changes in breathing patterns or shortness of breath

📝 PATIENT QUESTIONS

How can I slow the progression of my COPD?
Your COPD will get worse over time and medications may not increase your life span. However, if you do not smoke and you exercise and use oxygen therapy as prescribed by your doctor, you may be able to slow the progression of COPD.

What caused my COPD?
If you were a smoker, that probably played a major role. Other causes are pneumonia, tuberculosis, lung cancers, obesity, and alpha$_1$-antitrypsin deficiencies. Talk to your doctor to learn more about your specific cause.

Will I have to ever be on oxygen therapy?
Not everyone needs oxygen therapy. If the oxygen level consistently drops below 88% in your blood at rest or during activity, your doctor may prescribe oxygen therapy for you.

Will I ever need surgery?
If your symptoms get severe, your doctor may discuss surgery options with you. There are options, such as a lung transplant, bullectomy, and lung volume reduction.

What should I do if I feel my COPD is getting worse?
Be sure to tell your doctor immediately if you think your lung condition is getting worse, as this can prevent hospitalization. Know the signs and symptoms to be aware of so you can be prepared if your COPD worsens.

It is so hard to breath and my doctor wants me to exercise! Why?!
Exercise can improve the strength and the ability of your muscles to use oxygen. Eventually, you may be able to do more work with less effort, improving your quality of life.

Notes

Notes

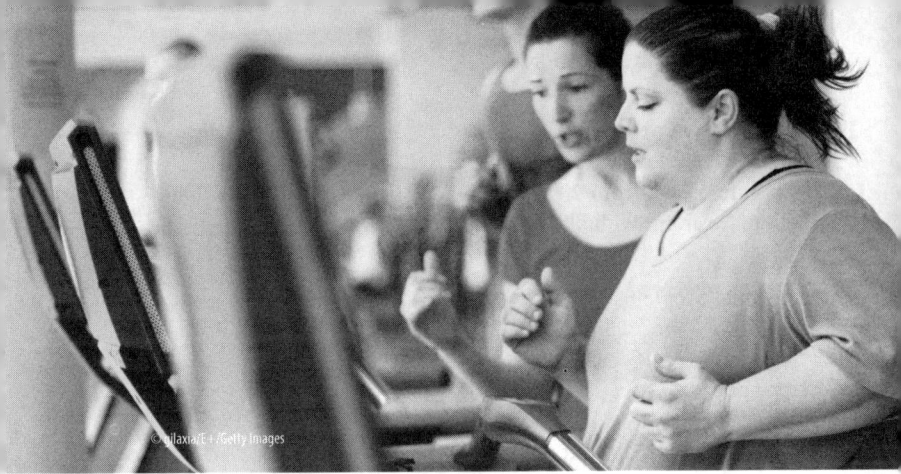
©Gilaxia/E+/Getty Images

CHAPTER 13
Obesity

▶ **Introduction**

Obesity rates range from 20% to 35% across the United States. Obesity can place an individual at risk for the following:

- Diabetes
- Hormonal problems
- Blood lipid abnormalities
- Hypertension
- Sleep apnea
- Joint problems
- Heart disease, stroke, and many other health issues

It has been estimated that healthy body fat percentages in adults should be about 26% for males and 30% for females. Obesity is most likely multifactorial, as an exact cause has not been defined. However, factors that contribute to obesity have been defined and are as follows:

- Excessive caloric intake
- Creeping obesity (i.e., high caloric intake, reduced activity, lower resting metabolic rate)
- Genetics
- Environmental factors
- A possible obesity gene

One common tool or indicator that is used to define ideal body weight is the body mass index, or BMI. To calculate the BMI, the weight in kilograms is divided by the height in meters squared, or one can divide the weight in pounds by the height in inches squared and then multiply by a conversion factor of 703. For adults, normal BMIs should be between 18.5 and 24.9. It has been estimated that 17% of children have a BMI greater than 30; this can result in many children being diagnosed with prediabetes. In adults, fat cells tend to hypertrophy or enlarge; however, in children, fat cells tend to multiply, a process called hyperplasia. Therefore, it is vital to stress the importance of controlling obesity at a young age.

One of the shortcomings of the BMI as a tool to categorize "normal or abnormal" weight is its failure to take into consideration the individual's muscle mass. For example, a short, muscular individual could have a high BMI and be categorized as an "overweight" individual, but not be "overfat." Other methods that are much more valid can be used to measure body fat percentage to accurately define and categorize lean mass. Hydrostatic weighing or underwater weighing has long been regarded as the gold standard. It involves Archimedes's principle of the laws of buoyancy (i.e., a person with more body fat will weigh less underwater and be more buoyant). One drawback or source of error using this method is that it requires individuals to exhale as fully as possible while completely submerged underwater.

A more modernized method that is quickly replacing hydrostatic weighting is dual-energy X-ray absorptiometry, or DXA. This method uses two X-ray beams of different energy levels to measure bone density and body composition. Another method gaining acceptance and popularity is the bod pod. The bod pod uses air displacement plethysmography (ADP) to determine fat and lean percentages similar to hydrostatic weighing, but the bod pod uses a very precise scale to measure body weight in a dry capsule. Other, more portable methods used in the field, but with less validity, are bioelectrical impedance analysis (BIA) and skinfold measurements.

Bioelectrical impedance works by measuring electrical impedance, which is the opposition to the flow of an electrical current through body tissues. This can then be used to estimate body fat percentages. Individuals should not be dehydrated, as this can result in an overestimation of body fat. The measurement is quite simple and can be taken by standing on a scale or with a hand-held device. Bioelectrical impedance is not very valid, but the results have been shown to be reliable or have a consistent error.

Skinfold measurements are considered more valid when compared to BIA. However, the accuracy can depend on the individual's measuring skills. Skinfold measurements require a hand-held instrument called calipers. Pinches of skin are taken at various places on the body and measured in millimeters. These measurements are then entered in an equation and body fat percentage is calculated.

Newer skinfold instruments use a technology called near-infrared interactance, or NIR. This technique uses an instrument or probe that is placed on an area of the body and emits infrared light or ultrasound, which passes through muscle and fat. This technology has recently become portable, but the accuracy is in question and is dependent on the technician's skill, as in skinfolds.

Fat can be stored in the body fat in many different areas. This can have an impact on health and is influenced, to a degree, by gender. The terms android and gynoid, apple or pear shaped, respectively, are commonly used. In android obesity, fat cells tend to enlarge or hypertrophy and the body fat is distributed around the waist, resulting in an apple shape. In gynoid or pear-shaped obesity, the fat cells tend to multiply, resulting in hyperplasia, and fat is stored below the waist, such as in the hips, buttocks, and thighs. Android obesity may pose a greater health risk when compared to gynoid obesity and has been correlated with a condition known as metabolic syndrome. Metabolic syndrome, or syndrome X, is referred to as a cluster of conditions that increase the risk for heart disease, stroke, and type II diabetes. High blood pressure, fat stored around the waist, and elevated blood sugar all contribute to metabolic syndrome. High intakes of refined carbohydrates are reported to be a major contributing factor to metabolic syndrome. With proper diet and exercise, metabolic syndrome can be reversed. Weight loss of 1–2 pounds per week is recommended to minimize the loss of lean tissue or muscle mass and lessen the likelihood of recidivism. Most of the weight lost during the first week of dieting is a result of water loss, and it has been estimated that as much as 70% of the weight lost during the first week of a diet is mostly due to a reduction in carbohydrate and protein intakes.

▶ **Medications**

A single medication used to treat or "cure" obesity has not been discovered. As mentioned earlier, one may never be discovered because obesity has been labeled as a complex disease with multiple factors. However, medications to treat obesity are available. In the 1990s, a popular weight loss drug prescribed by physicians was fenfluramine. Fenfluramine phentermine, or "fen phen," and dexfenfluramine were linked to pulmonary hypertension and heart valve problems and are no longer available. These medications worked by releasing a neurohormone called serotonin, which resulted in a feeling of fullness or satiety. Many of the weight loss drugs prescribed today work by either giving the individual a feeling of fullness or making it more difficult for the body to absorb fat. Patients who have BMIs in the range of 27–30, with health-related problems such as hypertension and/or type II diabetes, may be prescribed a weight loss drug by their doctor. Orlistat is commonly prescribed weight loss drug that is a lipase inhibitor, which means that it works by decreasing the amount of fat that is absorbed in the diet. Other weight loss drugs used to treat obesity are as follows:

- Lorcaserin (Belviq) activates a serotonin receptor in the brain to increase the feeling of fullness.
- Naltrexone/bupropion basically acts to increase the amount of adrenaline (norepinephrine), which may help modulate appetite and increase metabolism leading to weight loss. However, the effects are not fully understood.
- Savenda is an injectable medication that works like a hormone called glucagon-like peptide-1, activating areas of the brain to regulate the appetite.

Other, more-invasive methods used to treat obesity require surgery. Listed below are types of surgeries that can be performed in obese patients:

- Gastric banding (lap-band), reducing the size of the stomach
- Gastric by-pass, re-routing the small intestine to a small stomach pouch
- Bariatric surgery, removing a portion of the stomach

▶ Exercise

Both exercise prescription and exercise testing can be challenging when working with obese individuals. Many health organizations, such as the World Health Organization and U.S. Department of Health and Human Services, recommend that adults should get at least 2.5 hours of physical activity each week, and children at least 1 hour each day. Aerobic exercise at a moderate intensity (i.e., 50% to 70% of the Karvonen formula or heart rate reserve) is recommended to maximize caloric expenditure. Resistance training also may be included once an established aerobic exercise regimen has been implemented and should depend on the individual's abilities and goals. For most individuals, one to three sets of 10–15 repetitions or 65% to 75% of the one-repetition maximum (%1-RM) is a safe starting weight. To maximize caloric expenditure, obese individuals should exercise aerobically daily if possible, at a low to moderate intensity (i.e., 40% to 60% of the heart rate reserve). Aerobic activities should include modalities that exercise as many large muscle groups as possible, such as walking, stair stepping, or pole striding. Exercise modalities that support the body weight, such as stationary cycling and seated rowing, may be incorporated if the individual has joint pain or arthritis.

Many obese individuals are extremely focused on how much they weigh and check their weight many times each day. It is important to note that regular exercise will increase muscle mass and, because muscle is denser than fat, weight may actually increase if the same amount of weight as fat is not lost. To prevent frustration on the part of the obese individual, this may need to be a topic of discussion.

Often, it is necessary to exercise test an obese individual to determine fitness level and/or rule out coronary artery disease. Most exercise testing is performed on a treadmill; however, treadmills do have a weight limit, usually around 300 pounds, and may place uncomfortable stress on the joints. If that is a concern, an electronically braked cycle ergometer is the next modality of choice. Common problems that may be encountered when exercise testing on a treadmill include the following:

- Weight capacity of the treadmill
- The size of the examination table to prepare the individual
- Electrocardiogram artifact during the exercise test
- A large size or thigh blood pressure cuff may be needed
- Risk of orthopedic injury (many obese individuals have never walked on a treadmill, have difficulty seeing their feet, and are not aware of their body position on the treadmill)
- A controlled ambient temperature is desirable to prevent hyperthermia.

QUICK-REFERENCE EXERCISE TABLE: OBESITY

Frequency	Intensity	Duration	Modality	Warning Signs
Two to seven times per week as recovery allows	Rated perceived exertion (RPE) of 9–14 on the 6–20 scale	Interval/rest training may be necessary for some patients	Initially, treadmill or walking is the recommended modality	Report any chest pain immediately to the healthcare professional
Exercise may be performed daily to maximize caloric expenditure	Target heart rate intensities may not be appropriate if the patient is limited by body weight or joint pain	Aerobic exercise should be performed daily, if possible	Other modalities such as stationary cycles, rowers, steppers, and even arm ergometers can be applied. Resistance training can be prescribed once aerobic exercise reaches a continuous 20–30 minutes	Any sudden change in energy level, weakness, fatigue, nausea, or blood pressure changes
Exercise can be performed at home on off days	Exercise intensities or target heart rates at 50% to 70% of Karvonen or heart rate reserve (HRR) can be prescribed if exercise can be tolerated at that intensity	The goal for aerobic exercise duration should be a continuous 20–30 minutes, 5–7 days per week	Other methods of less-supervised exercise, such as swimming and aerobic dance classes, may be appropriate once aerobic times have exceeded 20–30 minutes	Rapid changes in breathing patterns or shortness of breath

✍ PATIENT QUESTIONS

I have a lot of fat around my stomach. Can I do sit-ups to "spot reduce" that area?
You can do sit-ups to tone the muscles at your abdomen. However, that alone will not burn enough calories to eliminate the fat from that area. Some areas for fat loss are more "stubborn" than others. Over time, expending calories will reduce your body fat in all areas.

How can I get rid of the cellulite on my legs?
There is really nothing special or different about cellulite, except in its appearance. It is still fat. You can lose it by reducing your calories and exercising.

Why do I even have to exercise? Can't I just use a machine that moves my body, like a toning table with a belt and massage feature, remain still, and let the machine do the work?
Those are called "passive" exercise machines. They do move your body and may help with flexibility; however, you are not burning enough calories to lose fat and tone muscle.

Why can't I just "burn off the fat" and lose weight in a sauna or sweat suit?
Saunas and sweat suits will certainly result in weight loss, but that loss will be water. As soon as you drink, the weight will come right back. When you sweat during exercise, it is because you are working and burning calories. Sweating prevents your body from overheating, but sweating in and of itself does not burn fat. Extensive time in saunas and sweat suits can result in dehydration, heat illness, and possible death.

I was told by my trainer that I should consider lifting weights as part of my exercise regimen. I don't want to become "muscle bound" and look even bigger than I already am, so what do I do?
Lifting weights and increasing your muscle mass will add weight. Muscle is denser than fat, but it also burns calories, where fat does not. Adding muscle will increase your metabolism and you will burn more calories, increase your flexibility and quickness, and tone up your body.

I am worried that if I gain muscle, it will turn into fat if I stop weight training. Is that true?
Muscle and fat are two different types of tissues. Without stimulation, muscles will deteriorate, but will not turn into fat. As you lose muscle, you may gain fat if you don't reduce calories.

I am a female and don't want to lift weights because I heard that weightlifting makes women muscle bound.
It takes a lot of work to gain muscle. Women do not have the same amount of the hormone called testosterone that men do, and will only gain a small amount of muscle. However, more muscle will make you look more fit, not masculine. The female body builders you may have seen on TV look very muscular because they have a very low body fat and many have taken steroids.

Notes

Notes

Notes

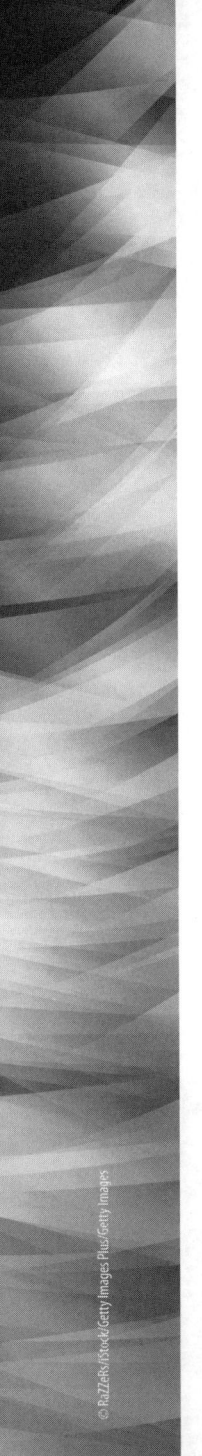

SECTION 3

Unique Exercise Populations

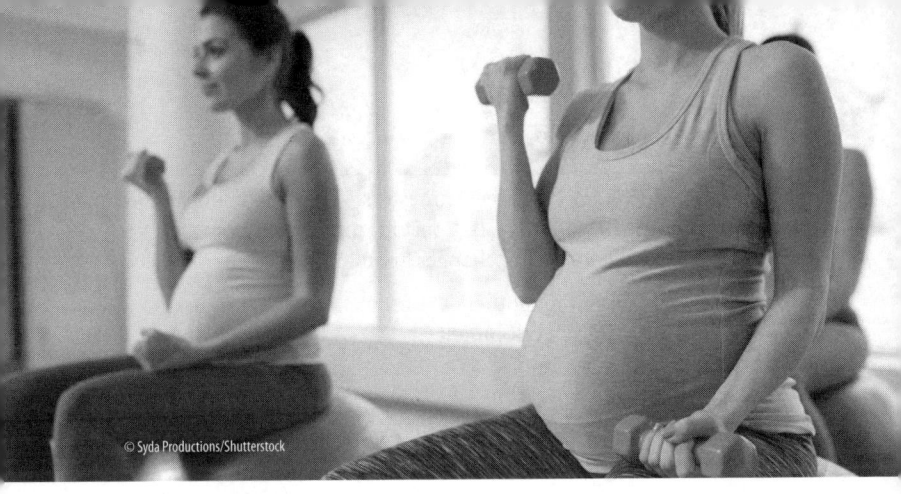
© Syda Productions/Shutterstock

CHAPTER 14
Pregnancy

LEARNING OBJECTIVES

Upon completion of this chapter, the reader will be able to:

- Define the three trimesters of pregnancy and understand how body changes during each trimester can affect exercise abilities.
- Be aware of additional vitamins and minerals that may be needed prior to and during pregnancy and their association with spina bifida.
- Define and understand generally regarded "safe" and "unsafe" exercises to prescribe during pregnancy.
- Know activities to avoid during each trimester of pregnancy.
- Know the benefits that can be achieved as a result of exercising prior to, during, and following pregnancy.
- Be aware of the absolute and relative contraindications that the American College of Obstetricians and Gynecologists has published and when exercise should be discontinued.
- Be able to prescribe exercise at the proper intensities based on the trimester and the patient's history of activity.

▶ Introduction

Pregnancy is divided into three trimesters. The first trimester is defined as the first day after the last period until the end of week 12. During this time, the following changes are taking place:

- Rapid weight gain in the mother
- Spinal cord and brain development
- Heartbeat
- Major organs begin to develop
- Hormonal changes begin in the mother

In the second trimester, weeks 13–18—or months four, five, and six—the gender of the fetus can be determined with skin and skeletal developments. The fetus has the ability to hear and sucking reflexes begin. In the mother, morning sickness decreases and stretch marks, joint pain, and swelling are common. By the third trimester (weeks 29–40, or months seven, eight, and nine), the fetus will gain about 0.5 pound per week. Fingernails, toenails, and hair develop and the eyes open and close. The fetus also has the ability to store minerals such as calcium and iron. The mother may experience contractions as the baby "drops" to prepare for delivery.

Note that, typically, maximal exercise testing is not recommended at any time during pregnancy.

▶ Medications

Any medications and over-the-counter supplements should be cleared by the physician or obstetrician. Folic acid is typically recommended prior to and during pregnancy to help insure healthy neural tube development and prevent spina bifida. Iron may also be prescribed.

▶ Exercise

In general, exercise during pregnancy is safe and does not put one at risk for a miscarriage. However, women who have not been exercising prior to pregnancy should not begin a vigorous exercise program. Physical activity may need to be modified or changed as the trimesters progress. Some examples of "safe" exercises during pregnancy include the following:

- Swimming
- Walking

- Stationary cycling
- Step/elliptical
- Low-impact aerobics
- Strength and toning exercises
- Pilates
- Racquet sports

Activities to avoid during pregnancy include the following:

- Contact sports
- Activities with a high risk of falling
- Scuba diving
- Sky diving

For example, during the first trimester, pregnant women should avoid excessive heat. Saunas, hot tubs, exercising in warm environments, and even high fevers that may elevate core body temperatures by even 3–4 degrees may be harmful. During this time, the neural tube is developing in the fetus and excessive heat, resulting in an elevated core temperature, could result in a premature closing of the neural tube, causing spina bifida.

In the second trimester, as the fetus begins to gain size and weight, exercises done in the supine position, such as the bench press, leg press, etc., should be performed with caution, especially with multiple gestations, to prevent any venous obstruction. The uterus may compress the descending aorta and inferior vena cava, decreasing blood flow and cardiac output to the mother and fetus. The mother also may experience postural hypotension episodes, resulting in dizziness.

By the third trimester, as the fetus grows, there is an increased need for blood and nutrients, causing more competition between the mother and fetus. Dramatic changes to the exercise prescription may be required during this trimester. As body weight increases, activities such as running, squatting motions, etc., may need to be modified to exercises done on machines that support the body weight. Elliptical steppers, rowing machines, and stationary cycles are but a few examples of appropriate aerobic equipment. There is an increased risk for hypoglycemia following exercise sessions lasting longer than 45 minutes, so snacks should be made available for treatment, if needed.

Other general considerations include the following:

- Avoid exercise during the hottest part of the day.
- Report any sudden weight changes or chest pain immediately.
- Keep a record of your exercise prescription to review with the physician if necessary.

- Avoid ballistic or bouncing stretching motions, especially during the third trimester, as joints become increasingly "loose" (known as laxity).
- Heavy weight training, or exercises involving a strong isometric component, especially during the second and third trimesters, is controversial and may result in vascular ruptures if Valsalva maneuvers or breath holding occurs.

Improvements in aerobic capacity and muscular fitness are possible to achieve during pregnancy. Furthermore, a better labor and recovery have been reported, along with an enhanced psychological well-being and permanent improvements in healthy lifestyle habits. Exercise also may result in a reduction in the risk for gestational diabetes and cesarean delivery.

Despite the fact that exercise during pregnancy is generally safe, it should be individualized to each mother. For example, the American College of Obstetricians and Gynecologists (ACOG) recommends that women who habitually engage in vigorous-intensity aerobic activity (i.e., the equivalent of running or jogging) or who are highly active can continue this type of physical activity during pregnancy and the postpartum period, provided that they remain healthy and discuss their progress with their healthcare provider. Despite these guidelines, the ACOG has published the following relative and absolute contraindications during pregnancy:

Relative Contraindications
- Anemia
- Arrhythmias
- Bronchitis
- Uncontrolled diabetes
- Morbid obesity
- Body mass index <12
- History of an extreme sedentary lifestyle
- Heavy smoker
- Poorly controlled blood pressure
- History of seizures
- Orthopedic limitations
- Thyroid problems
- Poor fetus growth

Absolute Contraindications
- Serious heart or lung disease
- Incompetent cervix or cerclage
- Risk of premature labor

- Persistent bleeding
- Placenta previa
- Ruptured membranes
- Preeclampsia
- Severe anemia

Exercise should be discontinued and the physician notified if any of the following occur:

- Vaginal bleeding
- Regular, painful contractions
- Amniotic fluid leakage
- Dyspnea, headache, and/or dizziness prior to exercise
- Chest pain
- Balance problems
- Swelling in the legs

Every mother has unique exercise abilities, and exercise history and desire should be evaluated in detail prior to designing an exercise prescription.

QUICK-REFERENCE EXERCISE TABLE: PREGNANCY

Frequency	Intensity	Duration	Modality	Warning Signs
Three to seven times per week as recovery allows	Exercise at 11–13 on the 6–20 rated perceived exertion (RPE) scale (50% to 70% of Karvonen or heart rate reserve)	Interval/rest training may be necessary for some patients	Initially, treadmill or walking are the recommended modalities	Any of the relative or absolute contraindications listed previously
Exercise may be performed daily, but should be adjusted to account for daily variations and trimester concerns	Target heart rate intensities may not be appropriate and RPE is now the recommended method for intensity	Aerobic exercise or other moderate activities should be performed at least five days per week for 30 minutes, if possible	Other modalities such as stationary cycles, rowers, steppers, and even arm ergometers can be applied. Resistance training can be prescribed once aerobic exercise reaches a continuous 20–30 minutes	Any sudden change in energy level, weakness, fatigue, nausea, or blood pressure changes
Exercise should be individually tailored, but a minimum of 150 minutes per week is recommended		The goal for exercise duration should be a continuous 30 minutes, 3–7 days per week	Other methods of less-supervised exercise, such as swimming and aerobic dance classes, may be appropriate; even activities such as general gardening and housework may be appropriate	Rapid changes in breathing patterns or shortness of breath

📋 PATIENT QUESTIONS

I have gained so much weight now that I am pregnant. I want to exercise to lose some of this weight!

If your body mass index before pregnancy was in the normal range (18.5–24.9), you can expect to gain 25–35 pounds. Exercise should not be done at this time to lose weight, but to improve your health and delivery.

Is it safe for me to exercise when I am pregnant?

In general, exercise during pregnancy is safe and does not put you at risk for a miscarriage. However, if you have not been exercising, you should not begin a vigorous exercise program. Physical activity may need to be modified or changed as the trimesters progress. Consult with your physician and a qualified exercise physiologist before beginning any exercise program.

What kinds of benefits can I expect if I exercise during my pregnancy?

Improvements in your aerobic capacity and muscular fitness are possible. Furthermore, an easier labor and recovery have been reported, along with an enhanced psychological well-being. Permanent improvements in healthy lifestyle habits may occur if you continue to exercise postpartum. Exercise also may result in a reduction in the risk for gestational diabetes and cesarean delivery.

What types of precautions should I take when I exercise during my pregnancy?

You should be aware of changes in your joints, breathing, and balance. Stay hydrated, minimize exercises that require you to lie on your back, have a snack handy, and avoid standing still or motionless for extended periods of time.

Will I need any type of special equipment to exercise when I am pregnant?

Depending on your previous level of conditioning, the most common types of aerobic exercises you will do during your pregnancy are walking and stationary cycling. These can be done at home or in a gym and do not require special equipment. If you are cleared for resistance training, most likely you will be using weight machines, which are available in most fitness centers.

How hard should I exercise during my pregnancy?

The intensity and type of exercise you do may vary depending on the trimester. A perceived exertion of 11–13 is recommended; however, as your pregnancy advances, you may find that you can no longer maintain this intensity. In addition, you may need to begin to use fitness equipment that supports your body weight as your weight increases.

Notes

_____

_____

_____

_____

_____

_____

_____

_____

_____

_____

_____

_____

_____

_____

_____

_____

_____

_____

_____

_____

_____

_____

_____

_____

_____

_____

_____

_____

Notes

Notes

_____

_____

_____

_____

_____

_____

_____

_____

_____

_____

_____

_____

_____

_____

_____

_____

_____

_____

_____

_____

_____

_____

_____

_____

_____

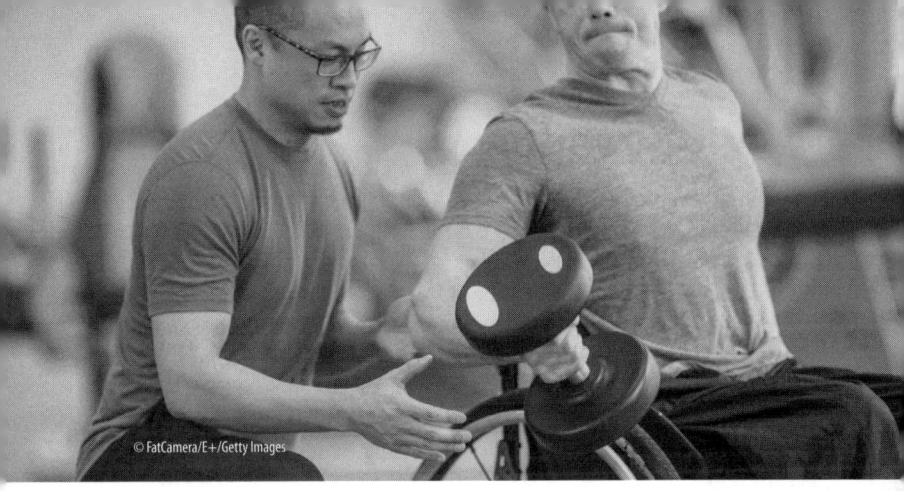

© FatCamera/E+/Getty Images

CHAPTER 15
Spinal Cord Injury

LEARNING OBJECTIVES

Upon completion of this chapter, the reader will be able to:

- Know the names of the different sections of the spinal column and how damage in each of the areas can affect paralysis.
- Understand the difference between tetraplegia (quadriplegia) and paraplegia.
- Know how complete versus incomplete injuries can affect paralysis.
- Describe emergency treatment measures for spinal cord injuries.
- Identify the complications common to patients with spinal cord injuries.
- Understand the warning signs and dangers of autonomic dysreflexia.
- Know some of the triggers that can lead to muscle spasms.
- Explain what the physiological responses are to exercise and how they can change based on the level of spinal cord injury and completeness of injury.
- Understand and show a working knowledge of how functional electrical stimulation, or FES, can be used to exercise muscles and the factors that can affect the treatments.

▶ Introduction

The spinal column is divided into different sections or vertebrae: cervical (C_1-C_8), thoracic (T_1-T_{12}), lumbar (L_1-L_5), and sacral (S_1-S_5). In most cases, spinal cord injuries at the level of C_1-C_8 or T_1 result in tetraplegia (quadriplegia), while spinal cord injury at levels T_2-T_{12} result in paraplegia. Injuries also may be defined as complete or incomplete, which would affect paralysis below the level of injury. For example, an individual with a very complete lower injury at the T_2-T_{12} level will have a complete loss of function below the injury level, but an incomplete injury may allow some feeling or function below the level of injury.

Spinal cord injuries are typically the result of a accidents, such as automobile collisions or diving in shallow pools, resulting in traumatic injuries. However, other medical conditions such as stoke, closed head injuries, multiple sclerosis, and muscular dystrophy can result in paralysis.

Unfortunately, it is not possible to completely reverse the damage, but measures can be taken to prevent further damage at the site of the accident or injury. Quick stabilization of the neck with a neck collar and transportation on a flat board to the hospital are necessary. Once in the hospital emergency room, maintaining an open airway, stabilization of the neck, and administration of steroids may reduce inflammation, reducing further damage. Other future and/or acute treatments may involve surgery to remove fluid and reduce compression (laminectomy) or traction to maintain a stable spine. Experimental treatment not approved by insurance, such using a hyperbaric oxygen chamber, in which the patient inhales pure oxygen, administered before or after spinal cord injury, have had some success.

Other complications and/or medical conditions that are common to patients with spinal cord injuries include the following:

- Decubitus ulcers (bed sores resulting from prolonged pressure on the skin, typically the buttock and hip area)
- Osteoporosis (brittle bones)
- Incontinence
- Pulmonary infections
- Autonomic dysreflexia, or a sudden increase in blood pressure (at T_6 and above)
- Reduction in cardiac output, especially at levels of damage above T_1

▶ **Medications**

Pharmacotherapy is often used to help with violent muscular contractures. Medications such as nonsteroidal anti-inflammatory drugs (NSAIDS) are used to treat chronic neurogenic nerve pain that often accompanies paralysis. Antidepressants may be used to treat depression, and antibiotics also may be used to treat frequent respiratory infections. Ditropan or oxybutynin may be prescribed to help with bladder incontinence; baclofen may be prescribed to help control muscle spasms and spasticity. After spinal cord injuries, signals that normally would reach the brain are sent back to the spinal cord, causing muscle spasms and spasticity. Common triggers include the following:

- Stretching of the muscles
- General movements
- Any skin irritation such as a bed sore
- Hot or cold contact to the skin
- A bladder infection
- A need to void the bladder

▶ **Exercise**

Exercise abilities and capacities can vary greatly in patients with spinal cord injuries. As stated previously, the level of damage and the degree of completeness are major factors. Exercise can be further complicated by a reduced autonomic nervous system response (sympathetic and parasympathetic). This results in little, if any, increase in heart rate (chronotropic response) and a lower cardiac output (inotropic response) and oxygen consumption (VO_2). Peak heart rates rarely exceed 120 beats per minute with labile blood pressure changes. This can be further complicated by the venous pooling of blood and hypotension, resulting in a reduced tolerance to exercise.

Patients with damage to the spinal cord at the T_6 level or higher are at the greatest risk and may be susceptible to a condition called autonomic dysreflexia. This results in sudden increases in blood pressure, as high as 175 mm Hg, and may be brought on by anything that can cause pain or discomfort below the level of injury. Signs and symptoms of autonomic dysreflexia are as follows:

- Pounding headache
- Goosebumps
- Sweating

- Stuffy nose
- Blurred vision
- Red, splotchy skin

If untreated, autonomic dysreflexia can result in stroke, seizure, organ damage, permanent brain damage, or even death.

An exercise therapy for patients with spinal cord injuries known as functional electrical stimulation (FES) has been used as a way to stimulate, and in some cases even increase, the muscle cross-sectional area in the lower extremities. Improvements in bone mineral density and cardiorespiratory benefits also have been studied, with improvements in cardiorespiratory function mostly reported when arm cranking is added to FES exercise. FES is not passive exercise and may be able to improve prognosis, reduce stress with activities of daily living, and possibly maintain muscle function and slow deterioration.

A common form of aerobic FES exercise involves applying a TENS unit to stimulate the gluteal, hamstring, and quadriceps muscles; this is coordinated by a computer, with the patient in a supine/sitting/cycling position. Aerobic FES exercise also may be performed in other positions, such as standing, depending on the level and completeness of spinal cord injury, and has even been applied to resistance training such as leg extensions. In patients with lower-level damage (typically T_5 and lower), hybrid FES exercise involving voluntary exercise such as arm cranking and FES-induced contractions of paralyzed leg muscles has been prescribed.

In order for FES to be effective, patients must have intact and functional lower motor neurons and the muscle fibers they innervate. Neurons are brain cells that transmit and process information by chemical and electrical signaling. The upper motor neurons in the cerebral cortex and brainstem relay information to the lower motor neurons, which then send signals to the muscles to contract and relax. If the lower motor neurons are damaged, the muscles will not respond to FES treatment. In most cases, the muscle fibers must demonstrate the presence of the stretch reflex and spasticity. Other factors that can affect FES-exercise treatments on a daily basis include the following:

- Bladder infections
- Respiratory infections
- Spasticity
- Decubiti (bed sores)
- Fatigue

QUICK-REFERENCE EXERCISE TABLE: SPINAL CORD INJURY

Frequency	Intensity	Duration	Modality	Warning Signs
Three to seven times per week as recovery allows	Exercise intensity can vary greatly depending on level and completeness of injury	Interval/rest training may be necessary and specific to each individual	Exercises involving as much muscle mass as possible should be performed to improve cardiovascular fitness and peripheral adaptations	Any of the contraindications listed previously
Exercise may be performed daily, but should be adjusted to account for daily variations in spasticity and possible infections or decubiti	Target heart rate intensities may not be appropriate for individuals with higher-level injuries, generally above T_1	FES-aerobic exercise should be performed as interval work/rest periods, with the goal to decrease rest times and increase work times to a maximum of 15–60 minutes	When possible, voluntary arm cranking and resistance training should be done to achieve fitness gains and may accompany FES-aerobic training	Any sudden change in energy level, weakness, fatigue, nausea, or sudden blood pressure changes
Exercise should be individually tailored to daily feelings	Rated perceived exertion (RPE) at 11–13 is preferred (50% to 70% of Karvonen or heart rate reserve), if possible	The goal for FES-aerobic exercise and/or arm cranking duration should be a continuous 15–60 minutes, 3–5 days per week		Decubitus ulcers, changes in spasticity, a need to void the bladder, rapid changes in breathing patterns or shortness of breath

📝 PATIENT QUESTIONS

Will I ever regain the feeling in my legs and/or arms again?
A full recovery is unlikely; however, depending on the severity and location of the injury, some feeling and function may return over time with rehabilitation.

Will aerobic FES-exercise allow me to walk again?
FES-exercise is not a cure for your spinal cord damage. It may help to slow your muscle and bone deterioration and increase your cardiovascular health if combined with arm cranking.

Why do some people with a higher level of injury compared to me have more function and feeling?
Generally speaking, high levels of injury result in more paralysis and a greater loss of function and feeling. It may be that the type of injury was less complete than yours.

What kinds of complications can I expect from my injury?
There are numerous potential acute and long-term complications that can arise that your doctor can discuss with you. Some may depend on your level of injury and how well you take care of yourself. Common complications include respiratory and bladder infections, rapid and drastic changes in blood pressure, pneumonia, blood clots, and fractures. Be sure to report any unusual symptoms or changes to your doctor immediately.

Are there any treatments or therapies that are successful in curing spinal cord injury?
Research involving stem cells, though highly controversial, has shown some promising results in animals. The treatment involves using stems cells to regenerate and repair damaged spinal nerves. More research is needed, as this treatment is still in the testing stages.

Are there any other treatments that can reverse spinal cord injuries?
There are other treatments, but not all of them may be appropriate for your level and type of injury. For example, a treatment known as epidural electrical stimulation applies electrical stimulation to the lower spinal cord to help restore function below the level of injury. Talk to your doctor to find out what treatment(s) may be applicable to you.

What are my chances of ever walking normally again?
That will depend on the level and completeness of your injury. With regular rehabilitation, some function may return; however, it may take a long time and lots of determination.

Notes

_____
_____
_____
_____
_____
_____
_____
_____
_____
_____
_____
_____
_____
_____
_____
_____
_____
_____
_____
_____
_____
_____
_____
_____
_____
_____

Notes

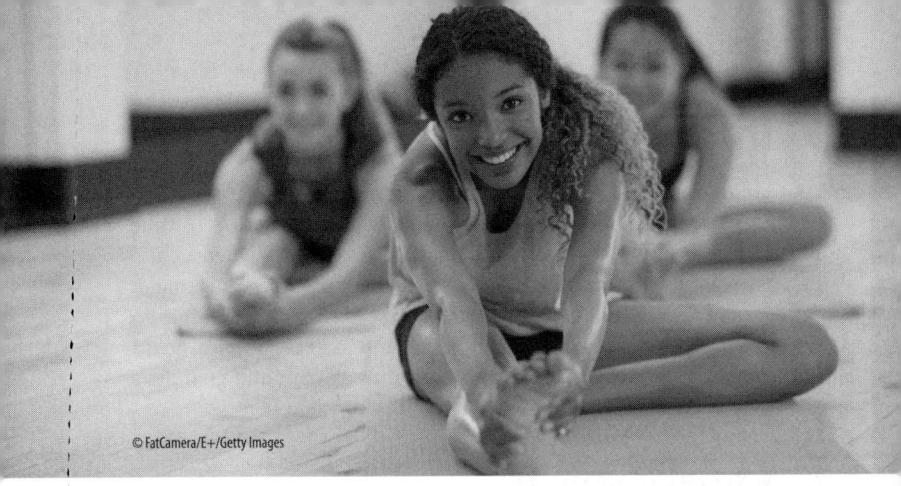

© FatCamera/E+/Getty Images

CHAPTER 16
Adolescence

LEARNING OBJECTIVES

Upon completion of this chapter, the reader will be able to:

- Understand why it is important to keep children well-hydrated during exercise.
- Know what types of exercise children are most likely to enjoy.
- Explain what the goal should be when exercising children.
- Define the different types of fitness tests that can be done to evaluate a child.
- Understand the pros and cons for using different modalities when a stress test is needed on a child.
- Understand the limitations that heavy weightlifting may pose on the long bones and epiphyseal plates.
- Identify the pros and cons involved when using free weights versus machines and how to progress a child when lifting weights.

▶ Introduction

As a child grows and begins to mature, many times the term "adolescence" is used to describe this development. It is the period of time following puberty, typically between ages 12 and19 years, when a child begins to develop into a young adult. Obesity rates in adolescent females have doubled since 1980 and, overall, adolescent obesity continues to rise. Programs offered to improve nutrition and increase physical activity have not been entirely successful. Educating parents and guardians is also necessary to improve environmental factors and success.

▶ Medications

In general, medications given to children do not affect their ability to exercise. Because Adderall or Ritalin are stimulants, they may increase the heart rate; however, children are rarely given target heart rates to follow when they exercise. If a child is on any medication, his or her doctor should be made aware if the child is engaging in any sport or exercise at any intensity.

▶ Exercise

Children can lose interest in exercise very easily. The challenge is to allow the child to choose from a variety of activities at different intensities and durations. In most cases, a child will choose a short-term, intense activity with a recreational component, such as basketball, soccer, football, roller skating, etc. The goal of exercise should not be to improve the VO_2, but to get the child involved in activities he or she will enjoy and is willing to participate in without complaining or lack of motivation. The following recommendations apply to all children.

Activities that are of lower intensity and more aerobic or endurance-like in nature will optimize caloric expenditure. Fitness testing usually involves skill-related activities such as flexibility, balance, and jumping tests. In some situations, a doctor may recommend a maximal exercise test to rule out concerns that may interfere with exercise. Children will usually perform and test better on a treadmill compared to a stationary cycle, as treadmills are self-driven and require less focused effort compared to a cycle. Children also may be predisposed to underdeveloped knee extensor muscles and localized leg fatigue on a stationary cycle, preventing them from maintaining the proper cadence.

Occasionally, but rarely, some children enjoy running long distances and some have been reported to even compete in marathon races. Children who decide to run marathons should be particularly conscious of the heat index; because of their immature cardiovascular system, resulting in a low blood-flow capacity to the skin, along with a large surface-to-mass ratio, they may be more prone to heat-related illnesses. This high surface-area-to-body-mass ratio also may accelerate heat loss in the cold, increasing the risk for hypothermia. When endurance training, allow plenty of time for recuperation to prevent overtraining. Similar to adults, it takes children about 10–14 days to acclimate to hot environments. Clothes that are light, with breathable layers that can be removed during exercise, are recommended. Cold fluids should be available at all times, especially during hot and humid days.

The notion that running will stop bone and joint growth in children and damage ligaments has not been proven, although limited research is available. Supervised endurance runs are not typically done in activity classes for children in elementary and junior high school physical education programs. However, many high schools do have cross-country running teams that may meet to run before and/or after school under the supervision of a coach.

Weight training, if supervised and performed appropriately, can be beneficial to any exercise program. Most children will be introduced to weight training in junior high school, possibly in a school gym that has a circuit or stations of different weight machines. The addition of lifting free weights such as dumbbells and barbells is usually more common in high school and applied to football players and powerlifting students. There are plusses and minuses to free weights versus machines. Competitive body builders and powerlifters typically use free weights in their workouts. However, both free weights and machines should have a place in workouts, depending on the goals. See **TABLE 16.1** for a comparison of these two weight modalities.

A beginning program for children usually involves two days per week and 10–15 total sets, performing 8–10 different exercises of 1–2 sets per exercise, with 8–15 reps, working both the upper and lower body muscles each workout. Power lifting, or heavy lifting at 90% to 100% of the 1-repetition maximum (1-RM) should be avoided because there is some concern that heavy lifting may be harmful to the musculoskeletal system. This may cause damage to the long bones and epiphyseal plates resulting in a stunting of growth.

Gains in strength will occur mainly from neuromuscular familiarization as opposed to hypertrophy, especially when testosterone is not fully adequate in the body. When 8–15 repetitions can be performed with a certain weight, the load can be increased for the next set.

TABLE 16.1 Comparison of Free Weights versus Weightlifting Machines

Free Weights	Machines
Better at improving total body balance and stabilizing muscles and core	Limitations to body size and core involvement
May require a spotter	Spotter not required
Loading and unloading of weight plates	Easy weight adjustment
Less room required (barbell, dumbbell sets)	Multiple machines require more space
Used in strength and size building	Weight stack may have limits on how much weight can be lifted
Can be more difficult to isolate muscles	Isolation of muscles can be easier
Requires more time to change weight loads	Workouts can be performed at a faster pace for endurance and strength

QUICK-REFERENCE EXERCISE TABLE: ADOLESCENCE

Frequency	Intensity	Duration	Modality	Warning Signs
Daily endurance or aerobic exercise if possible, or as recovery allows	Exercise intensity can vary greatly depending on age and level of conditioning	Interval/rest training that is specific to each individual with short rest periods	Activities involving large or compound muscle groups	Any signs of heat illness or dehydration
Exercise may be performed daily, and weight lifting can be added 2 days per week	Target heart rate intensities may not be appropriate for children	A total of at least 20–30 minutes each session	Recreational activities such as soccer, tennis, football, and basketball are examples of activities children typically enjoy	Any sudden change in energy level, weakness, fatigue, nausea, or sudden blood pressure changes
Exercise should be individually tailored to daily feelings	Rated perceived exertion at 11–13 is preferred, or no greater than moderate intensity	Aerobic, endurance exercise such as marathon training should allow plenty of time for recuperation to prevent injury and overtraining	Endurance running and weightlifting also may be added as described previously	Lack of interest or tiredness may be a sign of overtraining

🗒 PATIENT QUESTIONS

At what age should my child begin exercising?
If your child is interested in competitive sports, the minimum recommended age is 7–10 years. Once they reach this age, they can visualize and understand the concepts of teamwork and game strategy. Children of any age should engage in structured aerobic activities of 30–60 minutes each day.

What kind of activities should my adolescent child be involved in?
Adolescent children are old enough to get in involved in almost any sport or activity. Simple activities like jumping, climbing, throwing, and kicking can all be included in a more competitive and group sport, if desired.

How should I get involved in my child's exercise program?
Encourage your child, play with them as often as possible, and attend their sport events when possible.

My child does not seem interested in exercise at all! What should I do?
Don't force your child to exercise or use it as punishment. Try to encourage an activity your child likes, without earmarking it as exercise. For example, walk around the mall while shopping. Ask your child what they like to do and go from there with a light hand. Possibly incorporate their smartphone into an activity that gets them moving.

Is it safe for my child to do weightlifting?
Yes, it is safe, but the weightlifting workouts should be supervised by an experienced adult. Heavy, 1–3 maximum lifts should not be performed until your child is 16 years or older, typically high-school age.

What benefits can my child expect from exercising?
Benefits in children are very similar to anyone who is active and exercising. Improvements in cardiovascular and musculoskeletal health will occur. Maintenance of a healthy body weight and mental health are other benefits.

Notes

Notes

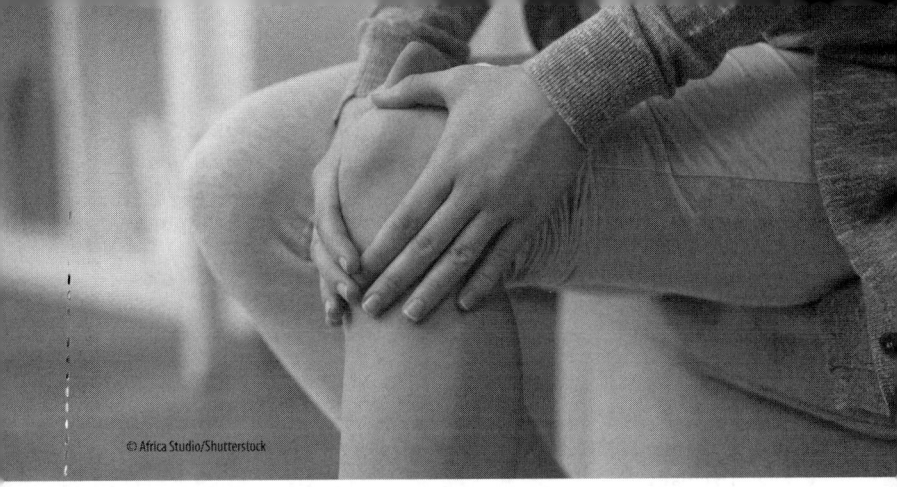
© Africa Studio/Shutterstock

CHAPTER 17
Fibromyalgia

LEARNING OBJECTIVES

Upon completion of this chapter, the reader will be able to:

- Understand the symptoms of fibromyalgia.
- Be aware of things that can trigger fibromyalgia.
- Understand the similarities and differences between chronic fatigue syndrome (myalgic encephalomyelitis) and fibromyalgia.
- Identify the types of exercise that may be beneficial in fibromyalgia.
- Explain the possibility of exaggerated delayed onset muscle soreness (DOMS).

▶ Introduction

Fibromyalgia is a disorder that is associated with widespread musculoskeletal pain and is associated with sleep, memory, and mood disorders. It is thought that the brain "amplifies" pain signals, causing constant pain and discomfort. It has been estimated that 5–10 million

Americans have this disorder; many are women between the ages of 20 and 55 years. The exact cause of this disorder is unknown, but it is associated with rheumatoid arthritis, traumatic injuries, and autoimmune disorders such as lupus. More specifically, reported symptoms include the following:

- Depression
- Memory loss
- Headaches
- Lack of sleep and energy
- Numbness in the hands and feet
- Muscle cramps
- Digestive pain
- Joint pain

Because many of the symptoms are common to everyday life, the diagnosis for physicians is challenging. In some cases, specific things, including foods, stress, and seasons, can trigger symptoms. Identifying, avoiding, or preparing for these triggers may help to reduce symptoms. Similar to rheumatoid arthritis, fibromyalgia symptoms can flare-up; there are typically exacerbations of the symptoms listed previously.

There is no cure for fibromyalgia; however, there are medications to help, which should accompany proper rest, exercise, diet, and stress reduction. Another disorder, chronic fatigue syndrome (or myalgic encephalomyelitis) has similar symptoms; however, chronic fatigue syndrome is mainly characterized by fatigue, whereas in fibromyalgia, the dominant complaint is musculoskeletal pain.

▶ Medications

Medications typically prescribed to treat fibromyalgia are antidepressants and antiseizure medications, including the following:

- Duloxetine (Cymbalta)
- Pregabalin (Lyrica)
- Milnacipran (Savella)

Some physicians also may prescribe acupuncture and other medications or homeopathic compounds that are not specifically for fibromyalgia, depending on the symptoms.

▶ **Exercise**

Aerobic exercise may help with some of the symptoms of fibromyalgia. Activities such as *tai chi*, yoga, meditation, and resistance training also may be beneficial. It is important to understand that many patients may have an exaggerated response to delayed onset muscle soreness (DOMS), especially during the first few exercise sessions. To attempt to minimize DOMS, exercises with a predominantly isometric component should be avoided, along with high-impact activities such as football or other contact sports. Depending on symptoms, exercise may need to be limited to 2 days per week for 20–30 minutes. Patients with more severe joint and muscle soreness should consider exercising later in the day, if possible. The health benefits of exercise can be similar to anyone without fibromyalgia.

QUICK-REFERENCE EXERCISE TABLE: FIBROMYALGIA				
Frequency	**Intensity**	**Duration**	**Modality**	**Warning Signs**
Two times per week initially, as recovery allows	Exercise intensity can vary greatly depending on symptoms and flare-ups	Interval/rest training may be necessary and specific to each individual based on symptoms	Exercises involving as much muscle mass as possible should be performed to improve cardiovascular fitness and peripheral adaptations	Any exacerbation of symptoms or delayed recovery time
Exercise should be adjusted to account for daily variations in symptoms and recovery	Target heart rate intensities may not be appropriate for some individuals due to daily variations in symptoms	Aerobic exercise should be performed as interval work/rest periods if necessary, with the goal to decrease rest times and increase work times to a minimum of 15–30 minutes	Resistance exercise should be a done as tolerated, preferably with machines to minimize chances of injury	Any sudden change in energy level, weakness, fatigue, nausea, or sudden blood pressure changes
Exercise should be individually tailored to daily feelings	Rated perceived exertion at 11–13 is preferred (50% to 70% of Karvonen or heart rate reserve), if possible			

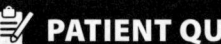 PATIENT QUESTIONS

What can cause my fibromyalgia to flare up?
Poor sleep, changes in dietary habits, and stress can contribute to flare-ups. Changes in weather, temperature, and even travel have been associated with flare-ups.

Can my doctor cure my fibromyalgia?
Unfortunately, fibromyalgia is a lifelong condition. Fortunately, it will not get worse over time, and will not cause an increase in damage to your joints, organs, or muscles provided that you do not ignore your symptoms.

Will fibromyalgia cause my death?
The pain caused from fibromyalgia will reduce your quality of life. Your risk of death from suicide is about 10 times greater than someone without fibromyalgia.

Can fibromyalgia shorten my life span?
If you ignore your symptoms, it can get progressively worse, causing damage to your organs and shortening your life span.

Is there a time during the day when my pain will be worse or better?
You may wake up with body pain and stiffness, which may improve during the day and then worsen at night.

Is my fibromyalgia a lifelong condition?
Yes, unfortunately it is a lifelong condition that affects your central nervous system. It is important to treat your symptoms and not ignore them to improve your quality of life.

Notes

Notes

Notes

Appendix A

▶ Methods for Prescribing Target Heart Rates

- Rate pressure product (RPP) (see below)
- %VO_2 reserve (The percentage of the difference between resting and maximal VO_2)
- %VO_2 (50–80%)
- % Heart rate reserve (HRR) (i.e., Karvonen) [(max.HR − restHR) × training %] + restHR
- % Maximum heart rate
- Borg rating of perceived exertion scale (RPE) (see below)
- The systolic blood pressure plugged into the Karvonen formula in place of heart rate

Rate Pressure Product (RPP):

$PRPP - RRPP \times (Intensity) + RRPP = RPP$ plugged in Karvonen

For example:
- 75 years old
- Max systolic blood pressure = 160 mm Hg
- Max heart rate = 145 bpm
- Resting heart rate = 80
- Resting systolic blood pressure = 110 mm Hg

$$232 - 88 \times 0.85 + 88 = 210$$
$$\frac{145 \max HR}{?} = \frac{232 PRPP}{210 RPP}$$
$$? = 131$$

TABLE 1 Borg Rating of Perceived Exertion Scale	
6	No exertion at all
7–8	Extremely light
9–10	Very light
11–12	Light
13–14	Somewhat hard
15–16	Hard (heavy)
17–18	Very hard
19	Extremely hard
20	Maximal exertion

Borg, G. (1970). Perceived exertion as an indicator of somatic stress. *Scandinavian Journal of Rehabilitation Medicine, 2,* 92–98.

Appendix B

▶ One-Repetition (1-RM) Chart

% One Repetition Maximum (1-RM)	# Repetitions
100	1
95	2
93	3
90	4
87	5
85	6
83	7
80	8
77	9
75	10
70	11
67	12
65	15

Case Studies

In the following case study, please choose the correct response from the options provided in parentheses.

▶ Chapter 2 Case Study

Kyle is a 48-year-old male with a family history of heart disease on his father's side. Kyle was diagnosed with a large heart attack 2 years ago, with a blockage in his (left coronary artery, circumflex artery). It resulted in an ejection fraction of (68%, 50%, 39%). Kyle has been feeling extremely tired lately and has experienced rapid (weight loss, weight gain), affecting his (face, arms, ankles and abdomen). Kyle's physician has increased his (beta-blocker, ACE inhibitor, diuretic) and recommended supervised exercise.

Kyle was referred to an (outpatient, inpatient) exercise program for supervised exercise 3 days per week with a minimum goal of (10–15 minutes, 20 minutes) of continuous exercise at an RPE of (12–15, 10–14) on the 6–20 RPE scale.

In the following case study, please choose the correct response from the options provided in parentheses.

▶ Chapter 3 Case Study

Many patients with a cardiac transplant have a history of (congestive heart failure, valvular problems). The most common type of heart transplantation is (piggyback, orthotopic). Jane, a 25-year-old female, has received a heart transplant and has been referred to you for exercise with no restrictions by her doctor. Jane showed up at your gym and wants to begin a weightlifting program. You decide to prescribe aerobic exercise at an intensity of (70% of the maximum heart rate, RPE between 10 and 14). Resistance training is also recommended at an intensity of (30% to 50% of the 1-repetition maximum [1RM], RPE of 10–14) to begin with. Her resistance exercise program should emphasize (strength, replacing loss of muscle mass). You should expect her aerobic capacity to be approximately (30% to 40%, 60% to 70%) of to normal. Over time, Jane can expect to (go off her medications, stay on her medications) as a result of her exercise program.

In the following case study, please choose the correct response from the options provided in parentheses.

▶ Chapter 4 Case Study

John is a 30-year-old sedentary male who presented to his physician with atrial fibrillation. He is otherwise free of coronary artery disease. John likely reported (chest pain and pressure, a thumping sensation in his chest and unusual fatigue) to his physician at a routine check-up. John's physician did an ECG and diagnosed atrial fibrillation; John was then referred to a cardiologist, who explained that atrial fibrillation involves the (SA node, coronary arteries). The patient underwent successful cardioversion and was cleared for exercise. John was referred to you for an exercise prescription. An appropriate exercise intensity could be RPE of (10–15, 50% to 85% of Karvonen). Resistance training for John (is, is not) appropriate. If John's atrial fibrillation returns, he should (continue to exercise until he sees his physician, discontinue exercise until he is cleared by his physician).

In the following case study, please choose the correct response from the options provided in parentheses.

▶ Chapter 5 Case Study

Ann is a 60-year-old female who has had a coronary artery bypass. Ann's doctor has informed her that she is not a candidate for any more surgeries and that there is no more that can be surgically done for her. Ann occasionally experiences chest pain when exercising at a certain rate pressure product; her angina is most likely (stable, unstable). Ann's exercise prescription intensity involves a target heart rate. Ann likes to use various types of exercise equipment and do resistance training. Ann should have (one target heart rate for all the various equipment, target heart rates specifically tailored to each type of exercise). The cool-down period for Ann should be (3 minutes, 5 minutes, greater than 5 minutes). Ann is most likely to take (beta-blockers, calcium channel blockers, ACE inhibitors or blockers, nitrates) to help with her anginal symptoms. If Ann experiences chest pain, she should (disregard it because her physician knows it is going to happen; take her medicine, discontinue the activity, call her physician).

In the following case study, please choose the correct response from the options provided in parentheses.

▶ **Chapter 6 Case Study**

John is a 46-year-old, relatively health man who is free of diagnosed or significant heart disease, with the exception of uncontrolled hypertension. John used to play professional football when he was in his 20s, but has been sedentary for the last 10 years and has recently received a mitral valve transplant. John's wife complains that she cannot always sleep with him because she is bothered by the "ticking in his chest"; this suggest that John has a (tissue, mechanical) valve. Because John used to play professional football, he can begin an exercise program (with, without) restrictions. John's heart valve will likely last for (10–20 years, his lifetime). John (will, will not) have to take his blood thinner the rest of his life. John's valve most likely failed due to (hypertension, rheumatic fever).

In the following case study, please choose the correct response from the options provided in parentheses.

▶ Chapter 7 Case Study

Paul is a 65-year-old man who was referred to your exercise facility by his physician for an aerobic and resistance training program. Paul has a DDD-type pacemaker. This type of pacemaker paces (only the right ventricle, both the right atrium and right ventricle). Paul has been given a pacemaker (with, without) the inhibited function. With the type of pacemaker he has, it (is, is not) possible to prescribe him a target heart rate. Paul wants to travel to see his grandchildren soon and is concerned his pacemaker will trigger the metal detectors in the airport. You tell him that his pacemaker (may, will not) trigger the metal detectors.

In the following case study, please choose the correct response from the options provided in parentheses.

▶ **Chapter 8 Case Study**

Mary is a patient in your exercise program and will be prescribed exercise between 50% and 70% of her heart rate reserve (HRR). Her resting blood pressure today was 130/80 mm Hg. Mary is classified as having (prehypertension, Stage 1 hypertension, elevated). She is more than 10% above her ideal body weight and her physician wants her exercise plan to be structured to maximize caloric burning. Over time, Mary can expect her resting blood pressure to possibly decrease by (1–2 mm Hg, 5–20 mm Hg, more than 20 mm Hg). Following exercise, Mary tells you that sometimes she experiences lightheadedness and that her physician is aware of it, but has not made any changes in her medicines. She should be advised to (continue to exercise as usual, extend her cool down by 5–10 additional minutes under supervision, increase her warmup time). Recently, a beta-blocker has been added to Mary's list of blood pressure medications. Because she has been following a target heart rate, she will continue to do so until she can have another exercise test on her new medication. Her target heart rate should be (decreased by 10–30 beats, remain the same, increased by 10% to 30%).

In the following case study, please choose the correct response from the options provided in parentheses.

▶ **Chapter 9 Case Study**

Joan, a 45-year old obese (BMI, 30), sedentary female with type II diabetes has been referred to you for an exercise program. Joan has been taking insulin injections for the last 2 years. You have Joan check her blood sugar on her first day prior to exercise; it is 90 mg/dL. Joan (should not exercise, should consume 15–30 grams of carbohydrate and re-check her blood sugar before exercising). Joan plans to exercise on the treadmill. The best place for Joan to inject her insulin before exercise is her (arm, thigh, abdomen). Joan mentioned that the last time she exercised, she felt a little dizzy and shaky. If this happens, Joan should (stop exercising and check her blood sugar, continue to exercise). Despite your best efforts, Joan continues to have hypoglycemic symptoms during exercise. Joan should (see her doctor, consume some carbohydrates and continue to exercise). Because Joan is obese, her aerobic exercise plan should emphasize (resistance training, caloric expenditure).

In the following case study, please choose the correct response from the options provided in parentheses.

▶ Chapter 10 Case Study

Martha is a 50-year-old female who had had type II diabetes for over 20 years. She was overweight as a child and was diagnosed with prediabetes. She has been feeling muscle cramping, fatigue, and shortness of breath with everyday activities. Her doctor checked her kidneys and they are functioning at less than 15% of normal. Based on these symptoms and tests, Martha (is, is not) a candidate for dialysis. Her doctor has advised her to begin an exercise program to help control her weight and improve her health. Martha has chosen to do hemodialysis at the dialysis center where you work. This type of dialysis involves (a tube placed in the abdomen, a dialysis machine). You are recommending a (stationary cycle, treadmill) for Martha's exercise. Her exercise intensity should be (high intensity with rest periods, low intensity with rest periods as needed). Martha should exercise (during dialysis, immediately following dialysis, right before dialysis). Because Martha is on dialysis, she (will need a kidney transplant as soon as possible, may do well on dialysis for many years).

In the following case study, please choose the correct response from the options provided in parentheses.

▶ Chapter 11 Case Study

PG is a 60-year-old sedentary, obese male (BMI 35) with a history of smoking, hypertension, and elevated cholesterol. He was referred to your cardiac rehabilitation program for exercise. PG has been diagnosed with peripheral arterial disease (PAD) symptoms at rest, based on the results of a (Strandness test, Bruce treadmill test). PG's doctor has asked him to get into a structured walking program to improve his walking ability. About (eight million, three million), new cases of PAD are reported every year in the United States. Individuals with PAD may suffer symptoms of (gangrene, blurred vision). In PAD, the (iliac, femoral, popliteal and tibial) arteries are commonly affected. PG's ankle-brachial index (ABI) at rest was less than 1.0. This ABI is (normal, abnormal). PG's doctor wants him to have a stress test before he begins exercising to rule out coronary artery disease. The recommended modality is (cycle ergometer, treadmill). Following the exercise test, the patient's primary mode of exercise equipment should be (treadmill, rower, arm ergometer). The ideal goal is to get PG to walk continuously for (5–10 minutes, 20 minutes, or more).

In the following case study, please choose the correct response from the options provided in parentheses.

▶ **Chapter 12 Case Study**

PJ is a thin, frail, catabolic man with a long history of smoking who has a rare alpha$_1$-antitrypsin deficiency. PJ has most likely been diagnosed with (emphysema, chronic bronchitis) and will exhibit a difficult time (inhaling, exhaling). He presents with a (moist, raspy cough; little to no cough). PJ will often have a (hypoinflated, hyperinflated) chest. The structures in his lungs that have been damaged are his (bronchial airways, alveoli). This patient has been referred to your cardiac rehabilitation program. Patients with COPD traditionally are placed in programs where they exercise every (Tuesday and Thursday; Monday, Wednesday, and Friday). PJ has been cleared for exercise in your cardiac rehabilitation program and instructed on the technique of pursed-lip breathing to help him (exhale, inhale) trapped air in the lungs.

In the following case study, please choose the correct response from the options provided in parentheses.

▶ **Chapter 13 Case Study**

Lisa is a sedentary, obese 50-year-old female with a BMI of (24, 27). Her doctor wants Lisa to learn to exercise in a structured exercise program, and she was referred to you. Lisa is prediabetic and runs the risk for (type I, type II) diabetes. Lisa mentioned that she had trouble sleeping; she most likely has (sleep apnea, an overactive thyroid). The weight gain that Lisa has experienced has occurred over the last 10 years. Lisa's weight gain is a result of (creeping obesity, binging on fried foods and ice cream). Her doctor has decided to put Lisa on a weight loss medication called Orlistat. This medication works by (stimulating the metabolic rate, reducing the amount of fat absorbed in the diet). Lisa also has been diagnosed with metabolic syndrome. She most likely has (android, gynoid) obesity. Metabolic syndrome, or syndrome X has been associated with a greater risk for (heart disease, low back pain). Her exercise program should maximize caloric expenditure; this is best accomplished by (daily, low- to moderate-intensity exercise; high-intensity interval training).

In the following case study, please choose the correct response from the options provided in parentheses.

▶ Chapter 14 Case Study

Lori is a 30-year-old, healthy individual with a sedentary lifestyle that does not involve regular exercise. Lori is worried that she will get "fat" during her pregnancy and postpartum, like many of her friends. Her physician has cleared her to exercise and she has joined your fitness center. Lori's exercise program should be (vigorous, light to moderate) to prevent "fat" gain. During the first trimester, Lori should be warned against (exercising in warm, hot environments; jogging). (Leg presses, Pilates) should be done with caution during the second trimester. During the (first, second, third) trimester, the exercise prescription may require the largest modification. The intensity for Lori's aerobic exercise should be set at (an RPE, a target heart rate). As a result of a regular exercise program, Lori can expect (minimal weight and fat gain, a better labor and recovery). Exercise should be discontinued and the physician notified if (swelling in the legs, vaginal bleeding, dizziness prior to exercise) occur.

In the following case study, please choose the correct response from the options provided in parentheses.

▶ Chapter 15 Case Study

Charlie is a 25-year-old male who was recently diagnosed with a spinal cord injury after he dove into a pool and hit his head on the bottom. Charlie's spinal cord injury was complete at the C_7 level. This would mean Charlie is a (paraplegic, quadriplegic). A complete injury means that Charlie (will, will not) have some feeling below his level of injury. After evaluating Charlie's upper and lower motor neuron function, it was determined by Charlie's doctor that his lower motor neurons were intact and functional. This means that Charlie (may, may not) be a candidate for FES-exercise. If a candidate, Charlie's FES-exercise would involve exercising the (leg muscles, arm muscles, a combination of both legs and arms). As a result of the FES-exercise, Charlie can expect (improved cardiovascular function, enhanced bone mineral density, improved activities of daily living, improved prognosis, reduced stress levels, slower muscle deterioration). (Bladder infections, Respiratory infections, Spasticity, Decubiti, Fatigue) can affect Charlie's ability to perform FES-exercise on any given day.

In the following case study, please choose the correct response from the options provided in parentheses.

▶ **Chapter 16 Case Study**

Rodney is a 13-year-old teenager who was diagnosed with attention deficit disorder (ADD) and placed on Adderall. Rodney has a body mass index of 30 and has been advised by a dietitian to lose weight. Rodney has been placed on a healthier eating plan, but his family doctor also has advised him to exercise. The best type of exercise for Rodney is (endurance training to burn calories, weight lifting to build muscle, recreational short-term activities). The medication that Rodney is taking (will, will not) affect his target heart rate. Rodney has decided to enroll in a basketball camp that will have many practices outdoors. Children are (more, less) prone to heat-related illnesses. Eventually, Rodney has expressed an interest in lifting weights. His weight lifting program should be (two, three, five) days per week.

In the following case study, please choose the correct response from the options provided in parentheses.

▶ Chapter 17 Case Study

Jody is a 30-year-old obese female with a body mass index (BMI) of 35 who has been struggling with fibromyalgia for the last 5 years. Her doctor thinks her fibromyalgia was triggered when she was diagnosed with (lupus, mitral valve prolapse) 5 years ago. Jody was advised by her physician to consult a qualified healthcare provider and begin an aerobic exercise program. Other activities such as *tai chi*, yoga, and meditation (may, may not) be beneficial. Jody's trainer advised her to exercise (two, five) days per week. Jody (should, should not) be given a target heart rate range and be encouraged to exercise at that intensity. The best time of the day for Jody to exercise is (morning, evening, mid-day).

References

Franklin, B. A., Gordon, S., & Timmis, G. C., (Eds.). (1989). *Exercise in modern medicine*. Baltimore, MD: Williams & Wilkins.

Leutholtz, B. C., & Ripoll, I. (2011). *Exercise and disease management* (2nd ed.). Boca Raton, FL: CRC Press.

Moore, G. E., Durstine, J. L., & Painter, P. L., (Eds.). (2016). *ACSM's exercise management for persons with chronic diseases and disabilities*. Champaign, IL: Human Kinetics.

Swain, D. P., & Leutholtz, B. C. (2007). *Exercise prescription: A case study approach to the ACSM Guidelines*. Champaign, IL: Human Kinetics.

Wegner, N. K., & Hellerstein, H. K. (1992). *Rehabilitation of the coronary patient* (3rd ed.). New York, NY: Churchill Livingstone.

Index